OVER 50 AND STILL COOKING!

Recipes for Good Health and Long Life

Edna Langholz, M.S., R.D.
Betsy Manis, R.D.
Sandra Nissenberg, M.S., R.D.
Jane Tougas
Audrey Wright, M.S., R.D.

BRISTOL PUBLISHING ENTERPRISES, INC.
SAN LEANDRO, CALIFORNIA

Printed in the United States of America.

ISBN 1-55867-005-X

Cover design by Frank Paredes
Cover photography by John Benson
Food stylist Stephanie Greenleigh

TABLE OF CONTENTS

About the Authors

Edna Langholz, M.S., R.D. is president of Langholz Consultants, Inc., in Tulsa. She has served as executive director of the American Dietetic Association Foundation and director of the National Center for Nutrition and Dietetics as well as past president of the American Dietetic Association and its foundation.

Betsy Manis, R.D. teaches nutrition at Tulsa Junior College and has promoted nutrition in supermarkets, health clubs, spas and the media.

Sandra Nissenberg, M.S., R.D. serves as consultant in the Chicago area after spending seven years on staff with the American Dietetic Association.

Jane Tougas is president of JBTideas, a Chicago-based marketing, communications and publishing firm. Currently she serves as editorial director of *Top Shelf*, a bi-monthly bar and beverage management magazine.

Audrey Wright, M.S., R.D. is administrator of the Father Walter Memorial Center in Montgomery, Alabama. She has served on the board of directors of the American Dietetic Association and as president of its foundation.

1. Prime Time Nutrition

You may be over 50, but there's no doubt you're still cooking—with energy, vitality and a taste for the good life. Mix these ingredients with some nutrition know-how, and you have a recipe for prime-time healthy eating.

Over the years you've learned that eating right can make a big difference in your health, appearance and well-being. As you move through the next decades, life's "prime time," good nutrition is more important than ever.

That's what *Over 50 and Still Cookin'!* is all about. It's not a "diet" book. It's not a book for people who require special or restrictive diets. Our goal is to help you develop a foodstyle you can live with and feel good about—a shopping, cooking and eating plan that brings you taste, convenience and, most of all, good nutrition.

Your Foodstyle

As we grow older, lots of things affect our food selection and eating habits. Taste takes on new importance, and most nutrition professionals agree that sensible food choices today can play a major role in our health tomorrow. If you're in your 50's or older, you should be able to look forward to more decades of the best that life has to offer. So, it's never too late to craft a foodstyle based on your lifestyle, likes, dislikes and unique nutritional needs.

Everyone is more health-conscious today. Diet advice floods the airwaves and fills column after column of your favorite newspapers and magazines. But what works for your neighbor may not work for you. The fact is that no one diet or food can work miracles. Your best bet is to make informed choices based on your needs and your food preferences. If you've fallen into some less-than-healthy food habits, don't despair—and don't try to change your foodstyle overnight. Be realistic.

An Action Plan

It can be done! But developing a healthy foodstyle is going to take some thought and planning. We've collected more than 100 recipes and tried to simplify some basic nutrition guidelines to help you find and achieve your personal best. We've also included quick tips on selecting and preparing some basic foods.

Maybe weight control is your concern right now. Maybe you're looking for ways to lower your cholesterol, limit the sodium in your diet or increase the fiber. You can accomplish all of these goals and still enjoy all the foods you eat—if you invest the time in assessing your needs, your tastes in food and the role your lifestyle plays in how you shop, cook and eat.

Healthy food can be good-tasting food. You don't have to give up old-time favorites to lower fat, control cholesterol, increase fiber or reduce sodium. In fact, you'll recognize many of the recipes we've included here. Some simple ingredient substitutions or adjustments in preparation style have made them healthier—and no less tasty. And because how a food looks can be just as appetizing as how it tastes, we've also offered you some ideas on presentation. Don't save these tips just for entertaining. Everyday foods should look "good enough to eat," too.

You might be shopping and cooking for just one or two people. Maybe it's hard for you to motivate yourself to prepare a variety of recipes—it's easier to eat the same thing again and again. Without some variety, though, you'll get bored fast and be tempted to break the monotony with convenience foods or by skipping a meal altogether. Avoid sabotaging your healthy foodstyle by preparing a wide variety of recipes in quantity, dividing them and freezing portions for future use. Most of the recipes in this book have been selected and adjusted with this in mind.

The Big Picture

Variety, moderation and balance are the cornerstones of good nutrition. Remember, just as no one food can work miracles, no one food can create disaster. Look at the big picture. For example, if one recipe or serving has a slightly higher-than-recommended value for calories, just be sure that the rest of your meal, or the other meals you eat that day, contain foods that are low in calories. Try to save your splurges for travel, parties or restaurant dining.

If one of your favorite recipes is high in fat or cholesterol, substituting a "lighter" fat, such as reduced-fat salad dressing, light mayonnaise or lowfat cheese, may bring it in line with your healthy foodstyle.

Adjusting serving size also can help you control your diet. Your favorite chocolate cake may be high in everything you're trying to avoid, but that doesn't mean you must banish it from your table forever. Cut your portion by half or more and save it for an occasional splurge.

Sometimes it's good for the spirit to eat a small portion of the "real thing," as long as you balance that choice with other, more nutritious foods. Gradually, you can learn to satisfy your sweet tooth with naturally sweet fruits. They're high in healthy carbohydrates and low in fat. Your favorite chocolate cake is not!

You Told Us

In order to help us decide what you wanted to know, we polled a cross-section of the active 50+ group. You told us that you want to know more about the nutrients in your food. You don't want to feel guilty when you eat, and you don't want to be nervous about nutrition! You want an authority who is *realistic* in helping you develop a practical, positive, and enjoyable 50+ foodstyle.

You told us that you love your old favorite recipes but are concerned because you think you cannot use them anymore. You watch your weight—or try to. You hear a lot about how cholesterol, fat, fiber, sodium and some of the vitamins and minerals can affect your health. What you need is a cookbook that can put it all together to help you lighten up the way you prepare your food.

You still like to cook, but not all the time. You still appreciate the taste of good food but want easy, quick health-oriented recipes. Many of you are looking for lighter recipes for entertaining because your friends are *also* concerned about what they eat.

You told us a lot, and we listened. But one message came through loud and clear: "Don't take everything we love to eat away from us."

So We Responded—Here's How to Use Our Book
Nutritional Analysis

We've included a nutrient breakdown for each recipe presented here. This information will be helpful to you in planning well-balanced menus that feature a variety of tasty foods. The nutrients we've specified per serving are:

- calories
- grams of protein
- grams of carbohydrate
- grams of total fat
- grams of saturated fat
- grams of monounsaturated fat
- grams of polyunsaturated fat
- grams of dietary fiber
- milligrams of cholesterol
- milligrams of sodium

Rather than using a single source, we used a number of sources to give you the most reliable information.*

We've also looked at *all* of the nutrients you need, especially those that are of concern for older adults. We have identified good sources of these vitamins and minerals. We have included this and other information about why we chose these recipes especially for you.

When analyzing these recipes, we made the following decisions:

- Meats are lean and free of excess fat.

- When a marinade or dressing is poured over

---

*
THE FOOD PROCESSOR II, ESHA Research, Salem, Oregon, 1988
FOOD VALUES OF PORTIONS COMMONLY USED, Jean A.T. Pennington,
    15th Edition, Harper and Row, New York, 1989
Nutrient data from food industries and manufacturers
RECOMMENDED DIETARY ALLOWANCES, National Research Council, 10th
    Edition, National Academy Press, Washington, D.C., 1989

a food, calculations are based on the amount absorbed, and not on the amount discarded.

- When preparing a recipe with an alcoholic beverage, the alcohol content is assumed to be burned off in the cooking process; therefore, the analysis does not include alcohol which has been heated. There may be some carbohydrate residue remaining which would yield a small number of calories, depending on the type of alcohol used.

- Ingredients listed as optional are not included in the nutrient analysis.

- If a choice of ingredients is listed, the first one is used in the analysis.

- When no specific type of flour or sugar is indicated, we used white.

In the nutritional information for each recipe, most of the figures have been rounded off. Recipes are written for people on regular diets. If you are on a special diet, contact a registered dietitian for assistance in incorporating specific recipes into your diet plan.

The recipes in this book can all be incorporated into a healthy foodstyle once you learn to balance your overall food intake. One serving from any recipe here contains no more fat than a 1-ounce ladle of regular Italian salad dressing or any other regular salad dressing. That ladle (2 tablespoons) contains 17 grams of fat and 159 calories from fat! Most people use more than this just on their salads.

We have told you how we adjusted our favorite recipes to make them healthier, but we have left some of the decisions to you by making suggestions about how you can further reduce calories, fat, cholesterol or sodium in many of these dishes.

Interspersed among the recipes, you'll find some pages that offer quick hints on selecting and preparing some basic foods like chicken breasts, fish fillets and soups. These tips offer a fast look at nutritious foods that are tasty and easy to prepare.

Symbols

We have included symbols as indicators of recipes which could be used if you are watching the fat, cholesterol, fiber or sodium in your foods. These symbols and guidelines were developed for the American Dietetic Association Foundation's *Dietitian's Food Favorites*. We are pleased that permission has been granted for us to use them in this book to help you select recipes for healthier dining. Just remember that the symbols refer to one serving and are not intended to suggest that the foods be used in unlimited amounts. Look at all of the foods you eat during the day to arrive at the proper balance of the nutrient(s) about which you are concerned. Remember the big picture!

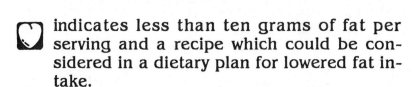 indicates less than ten grams of fat per serving and a recipe which could be considered in a dietary plan for lowered fat intake.

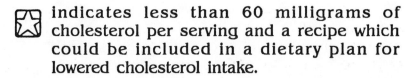 indicates less than 60 milligrams of cholesterol per serving and a recipe which could be included in a dietary plan for lowered cholesterol intake.

indicates two grams or more of dietary fiber per serving and is a good recipe to include in a dietary plan for increased fiber.

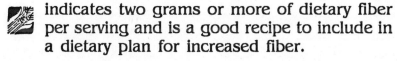 indicates sodium content less than 140

milligrams per serving and is a good recipe to include in a dietary pan for lowered sodium intake.

It's Your Choice

If you're looking for someone to tell you what to eat and when to eat it, you've come to the wrong place. We want to help you make the choices, help you develop and take control of your unique foodstyle. Remember, 50+ never looked better, never felt better. The 50+ years are prime time, time for you to safeguard your health for the years to come and time for you to enjoy the pleasures and benefits of good food.

2. What's All the Fuss About?

Cholesterol, sodium, fiber. You hear about these nutrients every day—in the media, at the doctor's office, at the supermarket. In fact, comparing cholesterol counts has become a part of casual conversation. Do you really know what these nutrients are? Here's a quick lesson.

Cholesterol and Fat

An important part of nerve and brain cells, cholesterol is made by the liver and also enters the body through foods of animal origin. Both forms of cholesterol contribute to your total blood-cholesterol level.

We need some cholesterol to stay healthy, but too much spells trouble. It gathers along the sides of artery walls and, over time, can accumulate to block blood supply to the heart and brain. Heart attack and stroke can result.

Without medication, you can't control how much cholesterol your body makes, but you can reduce the cholesterol you eat. Saturated fat can contribute to raising your blood cholesterol. Most saturated fats come from animal sources, such as lard, butter and meat fats. But some margarines, shortenings, and the tropical oils (palm and coconut), are also high in saturated fat. Monounsaturated and polyunsaturated fats are found in vegetable oils, nuts, avocado, seeds and olives; they are preferred choices.

Sodium

If you have high blood pressure or other medical problems, you may have been told to reduce the amount of sodium in your diet. What is the difference between salt and sodium? Salt is made up of two minerals, sodium and chloride. Salt is about 40% sodium; one teaspoon of salt contains about 2000 milligrams of sodium.

Fiber

Fiber is the part of plant foods that can't be digested. There are two kinds of fiber. Insoluble fiber (from fruit and vegetable skins and wheat bran) helps prevent constipation and assists in the treatment of many gastrointestinal disorders. It also may play a role in the prevention of colon cancer. Soluble fiber (from oat bran, oatmeal, dried beans and legumes, and many fruits) may help reduce blood cholesterol and assist in stabilizing blood sugar levels. Both types of fiber are found in most fruits, vegetables and grains, but in varying amounts.

Vitamins and Minerals

There are many vitamins and minerals that you need, and we have written more about them in our companion book *The Nutrition Game**. People over 50 often do not have adequate intake of vitamins A and beta-carotene, B6, B12, folate, C and D. Although iron, iodine, phosphorus, selenium and other minerals are necessary for your good health, it is not unusual to find shortages of calcium, zinc and magnesium in older adults.

*
Bristol Publishing Enterprises, San Leandro, CA 1990

Six Steps to a Healthier Foodstyle

STEP 1. Eat a Variety of Foods

No single food supplies all the nutrients you need, and no magic combination of foods will ensure your health and well-being. If you eat a variety of foods in a well-balanced plan, you'll usually get all the nutrients you need, including a wide range of vitamins and minerals that are essential to good health.

Age doesn't necessarily increase the need for vitamins and minerals; deficiencies usually occur because we just don't eat enough foods containing essential nutrients like vitamins A, D and C, as well as the B vitamins. An exception to this rule is the mineral *calcium*. Post-menopausal women may need more calcium to help prevent osteoporosis.

- Choose lowfat dairy products, broccoli, canned salmon and soybean products to boost calcium intake.

- Each day include dairy products, good protein sources, fruits and vegetables, breads and starches to provide the proper nutrients.

STEP 2. Reduce Fat and Cholesterol

Fat is a very concentrated source of calories. At 9 calories per gram, it supplies twice as many calories as protein or carbohydrate. Although the body needs a certain amount of fat, decreasing fat is the easiest way to avoid "middle age spread." Just because a little bit of fat is good doesn't mean a whole lot is better! Eating less fat, especially less saturated fat, is important because of the possible association between excessive fat intake and certain types of cancer as well as high blood-cholesterol levels.

- Keep calories from fat to 30% of the total calories for the day. This does not mean that each food must be limited to 30% of its calories from fat. We're talking about the overall fat intake from *all* the foods you eat. Some foods have little, if any, fat and can be balanced with those that contain more.

- To determine what your total intake of fat should be, divide the number of calories for the day by 30. For example, if you eat 1800 calories a day, your fat intake should be 60 grams. You can use the following chart as a guide:

Calories for the day	Grams of fat (30%)	Calories from fat (9 per gram)
1200 calories	40	360
1500 calories	50	450
2000 calories	67	600
2500 calories	83	750

- Identify the high fat foods that you eat and how much you eat of them. Begin to cut back gradually on the portions or make some healthy substitutions. It's too hard to change everything at once.

- Skip, skimp on or substitute for high fat foods. The amount of fat can be cut in half just by paying attention to amounts. Skip them entirely if you can. Skimp on salad dressing, margarine, oil, nuts or olives. Try substituting one of the new naturally sweetened fruit spreads for butter on your toast. Substitute lower fat cheeses for regular cheese, and use sherbet, lowfat frozen yogurt or ice milk instead of ice cream.

- Choose fats with the least saturated fat content, such as most of the vegetable oils. Avoid products with highly saturated palm and coconut oils. Only 1/3 of the total *over-all* fat should be saturated, and the other 2/3 should be equally divided between monounsaturated and polyunsaturated fats.

- Choose lean, well-trimmed meat. Select chicken and fish because they are not as high in fat as meat. Remove skin from poultry before cooking—that's where most of the fat is. Eight ounces of raw or six ounces of cooked meat, fish or poultry is adequate for the day.

- Limit cholesterol to 300 milligrams per day. Use egg yolks and organ meats less often.

- Skim fat from the top of soups and stews after they have been cooled.

- Use lowfat cooking techniques, such as broiling, steaming, poaching and baking instead of frying. Use nonstick cookware and nonstick vegetable cooking spray.

Healthy Substitutions

When a recipe calls for	use
whole milk	skim or lowfat milk to save as much as 8 grams of fat per cup.
cream	evaporated skim milk. It can be used in many recipes and it can be whipped.
sour cream	light sour cream or lowfat yogurt.
cream cheese	light cream cheese, 25% lower in fat.
mayonnaise	light mayonnaise or salad dressing.
shortening or lard	vegetable oils such as canola, safflower, corn, soybean, sunflower and olive.

STEP 3. Increase Carbohydrates
Emphasize complex carbohydrates and naturally occurring sugars and high fiber foods.
Complex carbohydrates are found in grains, starches, legumes and vegetables. Naturally occurring sugars are found in fruit and milk. These foods are good energy sources, are packed with a variety of vitamins and minerals, and fruits are often excellent

sources of soluble and insoluble dietary fiber.

- Carbohydrates should supply at least 1/2, ideally 55%, of daily calories.

Calories for the day	Grams of carbohydrates	Calories from carbohydrates (4 per gram)
1200	165	660
1500	206	824
2000	275	1100
2500	344	1376

- Cut down on refined and processed sugars such as table sugar and corn syrup.

You can boost dietary fiber to the recommended 20-30 grams a day by:

- eating unpeeled fresh fruit and vegetables
- eating boiled or baked potatoes with the skin
- eating whole grain breads
- using oats, oatmeal, cracked wheat and barley
- eating cooked peas and beans often (black, kidney, lima, navy, pinto, lentils, split peas and garbanzo)
- eating popcorn
- substituting 1/2 or all whole wheat flour in recipes calling for white flour
- choosing brown rice instead of white rice

Handy Food Fiber Guide

Food	Grams of Dietary Fiber
Cereals (½ cup)	
All Bran	13
Bran Buds	12
Bran Chex	4
Cheerios	1
oatmeal, cooked	2
raisin bran	3
Breads (1 slice)	
French bread	1
white bread	1
whole wheat bread	2
popcorn (1 cup)	2
Fruits	
apple	5
banana	2
grapes (1 cup)	2
orange	3
Vegetables	
broccoli (½ cup raw)	1
cabbage (½ cup raw)	1
carrot (1 stick)	2
celery (1 stalk)	1
cucumber (½)	2
green beans (½ cup cooked)	2
kidney beans (½ cup cooked)	7
lima beans (½ cup cooked)	8
pinto beans (½ cup cooked)	10
potato (1 small)	3
sweet potato (½ cup	3
winter squash (½ cup)	3

STEP 4. Watch Calories and Portion Sizes

Individual caloric needs vary from person to person, depending on age, sex, body type and activity level. As we get older, our metabolism slows down. That means we need less energy—or fewer calories—to fuel our bodies and maintain an ideal weight. Thus, it becomes increasingly important to choose foods with high nutritional value.

If you are overweight, you must reduce calories or increase exercise to shed those excess pounds. Portion control is one way to monitor calories. Eating smaller amounts of a variety of foods allows you to enjoy a wide range of tastes and textures.

- Beware of food plans that call for less than 1200 calories per day. You may not be able to get all the nutrients you need from such a limited food intake.

- Resign from the "Clean Your Plate" Club. Watch the amount, as well as the kind, of food you eat. It's easy to get twice the calories you *think* you're eating just by having second helpings or not watching the size of your servings.

- When you're cooking, refrain from adding that little bit of extra oil or margarine to the pan or using just a little more salad dressing when you toss. Those calories add up fast.

STEP 5. Limit Alcohol

If you drink, do so in moderation. Excessive alcohol consumption can be harmful to your health by contributing to several chronic diseases and affecting the way you feel.

- Alcohol will add calories to your diet but the

nutritional value is insignificant. Calories will vary between 70 and 150 per drink. Sweetened drink mixes add extra calories. Even tonic water has calories. For a quick rough estimate, add 120 calories for each drink or glass of wine.

- Limit your intake of alcohol to two drinks a day.

- Wine or other alcohol can be used in cooking as a marinade or for flavor. Most of the calories are burned off during the cooking process. A few carbohydrate calories remain, depending on the alcohol used.

STEP 6. Use Sodium in Moderation

Salt, like fat, imparts a lot of the flavor in food that we have become used to over the years. Although sodium is an essential mineral, too much sodium in your diet is not recommended.

- Limit sodium intake to 3000 milligrams per day.

- A food labeled "sodium free" will have 5 milligrams of sodium or less per serving; "very low sodium," less than 35 milligrams; and "Low sodium," 140 milligrams.

- Use fresh or frozen vegetables rather than canned. The difference in sodium may be as much as 300 milligrams! One half cup of fresh green beans contains 3 milligrams of sodium while the same amount of canned contains 319 milligrams.

- Use spices and herbs to replace the flavor of salt. If your recipe calls for garlic salt, use fresh garlic or garlic powder. Salt-free herb mixes, such as **All-Purpose Herb Mix**, page 55, can be used in place of salt or seasoned salt. There are "lite" salts available that have as much as 75% less salt than the regular seasoning salts.

• Cut the salt called for in a recipe by half or use just a pinch instead of a teaspoon to greatly reduce sodium in your recipes.

• Try a low sodium soy sauce for a tremendous sodium savings. One brand we found had 130 milligrams per teaspoon as compared with about 300 milligrams for the regular soy sauce. You can also water down regular soy sauce and still get the flavor.

• Use homemade broth (**Basic Beef or Chicken Broth**, page 46) to make your own soups. They will be much lower in sodium than canned soups.

• Select natural cheese such as cheddar (176 milligrams of sodium per ounce) or Swiss (74 milligrams per ounce) in preference to American processed cheese at 406 milligrams of sodium per ounce. Part skim ricotta beats cottage cheese—it contains 152 milligrams of sodium compared to 457 milligrams for ½ cup of cottage cheese.

• Limit processed and cured meats like hot dogs and cold cuts because they are very high in sodium. Fresh pork, beef, chicken and turkey are better choices.

• Watch potato chips and other salty snacks. The sodium content varies. Unsalted popcorn has 1 milligram of sodium per cup while buttered and salted popcorn contains 175 milligrams. One ounce of potato chips has 285 milligrams of sodium.

- Make your own salad dressing with oil, vinegar and your favorite herbs. It will have less sodium than commercial counterparts.

- There may be hidden sodium in the foods you use. Read labels and watch for any word or combination of words that say salt, soda or sodium.

Shake the salt habit—both in cooking and at the table. Give yourself a little time. You'll find your taste will adjust, and you won't even like the salty taste any more.

3. Appetizers

Artichoke Squares

64 squares

⬚ ⬚ ⬚ *These are easy to make ahead and freeze. They do contain some eggs but the cholesterol content is very low, since the four eggs are divided into 64 portions. This recipe encourages the practice of sautéing in just one teaspoon of oil. Part-skim mozzarella is lower in fat than Swiss or cheddar.*

⅓ cup chopped onion
1 clove minced garlic
1 tsp. vegetable oil
4 eggs, beaten
1 (14 oz.) can artichoke hearts, drained, chopped
¼ cup bread crumbs
½ lb. part-skim mozzarella cheese, shredded
2 tbs. chopped fresh parsley
¼ tsp. oregano
¼ tsp. basil
⅛ tsp. pepper

Sauté onion and garlic in oil. Combine remaining ingredients. Add onion and garlic; mix thoroughly. Pour mixture into a greased 8" square pan. Bake at 325° for 30 minutes. Cut into 1" squares and serve warm or at room temperature.

Nutritional information per square   17 calories, 1 g protein, 1 g carbohydrate, 1 g total fat, .5 g saturated fat, .3 g monounsaturated fat, .1 g polyunsaturated fat, 15 mg cholesterol, .2 g dietary fiber, 25 mg sodium

Mexican Bean Dip

*Who said dips had to be full of sour cream and fat? Kidney beans are one of the best sources of soluble fiber—and only 2 tablespoons will give you 4 grams of fiber, a lot for such a tiny amount. This dip also contributes iron and folate. It freezes well. Serve it with **Guilt-Free Tortilla Chips**, page 26, or pita bread.*

> 1½ cups kidney, pinto or black beans, cooked or canned, drained
> ¼ cup tomato paste
> 2 tsp. red wine vinegar
> 2 tsp. chili powder
> ½ tsp. cumin
> ¼ tsp. garlic powder
> 2 tbs. chopped green onions

In a food processor or blender, puree beans until smooth. Transfer to a medium bowl and add remaining ingredients. Mix well.

Nutritional information per 2-tablespoon serving   49 calories, 3 g protein, 9 g carbohydrate, .3 g total fat, .1 g saturated fat, .1 g monounsaturated fat, .2 g polyunsaturated fat, 0 mg cholesterol, 4 g dietary fiber, 179 mg sodium

Five Ways to Use Fresh Vegetables as Appetizers

Fresh vegetables are a "fast food" requiring little or no preparation. Their color, texture and shape make them appetizing to the eye, and that fresh taste can't be beat. With some care in handling and presentation, an assortment of fresh vegetables makes an appetizer that's lovely to look at and healthy to eat.

- Select only the freshest produce and store it in the refrigerator.

- Just wash and trim these:
  cherry tomatoes
  radishes
  mushrooms
  endive

- Cut these in slices or strips:
  cucumbers
  yellow and green zucchini squash
  red and green peppers
  celery
  carrots
  scallions

- Blanch these to bring out their color and flavor: (Vegetables require varying amounts of blanching time to make them tender, yet crisp. Microwaving is a quick way to blanch.)
  asparagus
  green beans
  broccoli

carrots
snow peas
Brussels sprouts
cauliflower

- Group similar vegetables together with 3 to 4 different types on each tray. Display them in baskets or in vegetable bowls like hollowed-out pumpkins, squashes, cabbages or peppers. Bowls made from vegetables also serve as wonderful dip containers.

Guilt-Free Tortilla Chips

16 chips

Love chips but hate the fat that goes with them? Corn tortillas are practically fat free, high in complex carbohydrates and a good source of calcium. These chips have 80% less fat than regular corn chips and are great with bean dip or as a base for nachos. No one can just eat one!

4 corn tortillas
nonstick cooking spray
1/8 tsp. paprika
1/8 tsp. cayenne pepper
1/8 tsp. cumin
1/8 tsp. garlic powder
1/8 tsp. chili powder

Spray corn tortillas with nonstick cooking spray. Sprinkle with spices. Stack tortillas on top of each other and cut into fourths. Place chips in one layer on a cookie sheet and broil 5 minutes or until crisp. Store in an air-tight container to keep crisp and fresh.

Nutritional information per chip   16 calories, .5 g protein, 3 g carbohydrate, .3 g total fat, 0 g saturated fat, .1 g monounsaturated fat, .1 g polyunsaturated fat, 0 mg cholesterol, .6 g dietary fiber, .5 mg sodium

Onion Sticks

Make your own onion bread sticks from whole wheat bread. This tasty recipe contains some fat, so pair it with a lowfat food like a salad or soup. Choose a heart-healthy margarine with high amounts of polyunsaturated and monounsaturated fat. Check the margarine label! The first ingredient listed should be a liquid oil such as corn, sunflower, safflower or soybean to assure that it is low in saturated fat.

½ cup softened margarine
½ pkg. dry onion soup mix
12 slices whole wheat bread,
   crusts removed

Blend softened margarine with soup mix until it is the consistency of a spread. Spread each bread slice with mixture. Cut each slice of bread into three strips and place strips on a baking sheet. Bake at 300° for 1 hour or until bread sticks are crisp. Serve warm.

Nutritional information per stick   46 calories, 1 g protein, 4 g carbohydrate, 3 g total fat, 1 g saturated fat, 1 g monounsaturated fat, 1 g polyunsaturated fat, 0 mg cholesterol, 1 g dietary fiber, 98 mg sodium

Hot Salmon Dip

Servings: 20

◯ ✩ ⊠ *These ingredients can be shaped into a ball and served cold rather than baked. **Hot Salmon Dip** is an example of a high-fat food that can turn out to be lower in fat overall when eaten with fresh vegetables and lowfat crackers. And remember that an appetizer is not a feast!*

1 (7¾ oz.) can boneless salmon, drained
8 oz. cream cheese, softened
2 tbs. chopped onion
1 tbs. lowfat milk
¾ tsp. horseradish
¼ tsp. dill weed
¼ tsp. pepper
½ cup slivered almonds

Combine all ingredients except almonds. Mix well. Spoon mixture into an oven-proof dish. Sprinkle ½ almonds on top of mixture. Bake at 375° for 10 minutes. Sprinkle remaining almonds on top.

Nutritional information per 1-tablespoon serving   69 calories, 3 g protein, 1 g carbohydrate, 6 g total fat, 3 g saturated fat, 2 g monounsaturated fat, 1 g polyunsaturated fat, 18 mg cholesterol, .3 g dietary fiber, 95 mg sodium

Hot Shrimp Canapes

48 canapes

◯ ✦ ✉ *The ingredients may look sinful, but the calories for one canape are less than a chip with dip. To lighten up and reduce calories, cut canapes into six or eight servings instead of four and use light cream cheese. The advantage of this recipe is that the canapes can be frozen uncooked and heated when unexpected guests arrive.*

8 oz. cream cheese, softened
1 (4½ oz.) can small shrimp
½ tsp. garlic powder
2 tsp. dried chives
12 slices white bread, crusts removed

Mash softened cream cheese with shrimp, garlic powder and chives. Spread each bread slice with 4 tsp. of the mixture. Cut bread into 4 portions (squares or triangles) and bake for immediate use or freeze for future use. Bake fresh canapes at 350° for 5 minutes or frozen canapes at 350° for 10 minutes.

Nutritional information per canape   39 calories, 2 g protein, 4 g carbohydrate, 2 g total fat, 1 g saturated fat, 1 g monounsaturated fat, .1 g polyunsaturated fat, 10 mg cholesterol, .1 g dietary fiber, 54 mg sodium

Hot Tuna Canapes

48 canapes

◖◗ ✶ ✶ Since these are cream-cheese based, you'll probably want to eat them in moderation along with some lowfat nibbles, such as raw vegetables. Substitute light cream cheese to reduce fat by 25%. Quick and easy!

    8 oz. cream cheese, softened
    1 (6½ oz.) can water-packed tuna,
       drained
    1 tsp. curry powder
    12 slices white bread, crusts removed

Mash softened cream cheese with tuna and curry powder. Spread each bread slice with 4 tsp. of mixture. Cut bread into 4 portions (squares or triangles) and bake for immediate use or freeze for future use. Bake fresh canapes at 350° for 5 minutes or frozen canapes at 350° for 10 minutes.

Nutritional information per canape   40 calories, 2 g protein, 4 g carbohydrate, 2 g total fat, 1 g saturated fat, 1 g monounsaturated fat, 0 g polyunsaturated fat, 7 mg cholesterol, .1 g dietary fiber, 64 mg sodium

Sausage Pinwheels

52 pinwheels

The original recipe called for pork sausage and pie crust. We "defatted" the recipe by using turkey sausage and biscuit dough. Tasty morsels at 16 calories per pinwheel!

1 can buttermilk biscuits (10 biscuits)
⅓ cup (3 oz.) bulk turkey sausage, uncooked, room temperature

Remove biscuits from can and combine into a ball of dough. Roll into a rectangle about ¼" thick. Spread turkey sausage evenly over dough. Roll long side of dough as if making a jelly roll. Slice with a sharp knife into ¼" slices. Place each slice on a non-stick baking sheet and bake at 350° for 15 minutes or until pinwheels become light brown. Serve warm.

Nutritional information per pinwheel 16 calories, 1 g protein, 2 g carbohydrate, .6 g total fat, .2 g saturated fat, .3 g monounsaturated fat, 0 g polyunsaturated fat, 1.5 mg cholesterol, 0 g dietary fiber, 59 mg sodium

4. Breads

Old-Fashioned Corn Bread 33
Pumpkin Bran Muffins 34
Our Favorite Bran Muffins 35
Four-Grain Biscuits 36
Applesauce Raisin Muffins 37
Popovers 38
Raspberry Coffee Cake 39
Strawberry Bread 40
Banana Bread 41
No-Oil Spice Bread 42
Wheat Germ Bread 43
Swedish Oven Pancake 44

Old-Fashioned Corn Bread

Go for the grain with this excellent source of complex carbohydrate. Serve with a bowl of pinto beans or other beans for a meatless meal that still gives you a complete source of protein without much fat and cholesterol.

2 cups cornmeal
2 tsp. baking powder
1 tsp. baking soda
1 tbs. honey
2 tbs. wheat germ (optional)
1 egg
1 cup buttermilk
2 tbs. vegetable oil

Combine all ingredients. Pour into a greased 8"x 8" baking dish or 12 greased muffin tins. Bake at 400° for 25 to 30 minutes or until brown.

Nutritional information per serving   124 calories, 3 g protein, 21 g carbohydrate, 3 g total fat, 1 g saturated fat, 1 g monounsaturated fat, 1 g polyunsaturated fat, 18 mg cholesterol, 2 g dietary fiber, 151 mg sodium

Pumpkin Bran Muffins

12 muffins

Hop on the bran wagon and enjoy these moist muffins. The pumpkin is one of those deep yellow vitamin A and beta-carotene vegetables, so there's lots of nutrition mileage in this recipe. Low in fat and high in fiber, it's so good you won't want to add butter or margarine.

1/4 cup boiling water
3/4 cup all-bran cereal
1/2 cup buttermilk
1/4 cup brown sugar
2 tbs. vegetable oil
1 egg
3/4 cup canned pumpkin
2 tbs. frozen orange juice concentrate
1 cup whole wheat flour
1 tsp. baking soda
1/2 tsp. pumpkin pie spice
1/2 tsp. allspice
1 tbs. dark molasses

Pour boiling water over cereal. Stir and set aside to cool. Stir together buttermilk, brown sugar and oil. Add egg and beat well. Add pumpkin and orange juice concentrate. Mix in flour, baking soda and spices. Combine two mixtures. Add molasses and stir until just moistened. (Batter will not be completely smooth.) Pour batter into 12 greased muffin tins. Bake at 425° for 15 to 20 minutes.

Nutritional information per muffin 108 calories, 3 g protein, 19 g carbohydrate, 3 g total fat, .5 g saturated fat, 1 g monounsaturated fat, 1.5 g polyunsaturated fat, 18 mg cholesterol, 3 g dietary fiber, 150 mg sodium

Our Favorite Bran Muffins

40 muffins

We have included this delicious muffin recipe because the batter keeps in your refrigerator up to 6 weeks. What a great way to prepare hot, homemade muffins anytime! Also try adding raisins, dates, or nuts for a different taste and the addition of a little iron in your diet.

1 cup bran flakes
1 cup boiling water
½ cup vegetable shortening
1¼ cups sugar
½ tsp. salt
2 beaten eggs
2 cups buttermilk
2 cups all-bran cereal
2½ cups flour
1 tbs. baking soda
1 tsp. vanilla

Combine bran flakes with boiling water. Let cool. Cream shortening and sugar. Add remaining ingredients and stir in bran-water mixture. Store batter in glass jars in refrigerator until ready to bake. Pour batter into greased muffin tins and bake at 375° for 20 minutes or until muffins test done.

Nutritional information per muffin 97 calories, 2 g protein, 17 g carbohydrate, 3 g total fat, 1 g saturated fat, 1 g monounsaturated fat, 1 g polyunsaturated fat, 11 mg cholesterol, 2 g dietary fiber, 162 mg sodium

Four-Grain Biscuits

24 small biscuits

Instead of buying biscuit mix, make this mix ahead and store it in the refrigerator. These biscuits contain many good sources of fiber and are a good way to include oats and other whole grains in your diet.

2 cups flour
2 cups whole wheat flour
¾ cup nonfat dry milk powder
½ cup uncooked oats (or oat bran)
½ cup cornmeal
3 tbs. baking powder
1 cup margarine
2 tbs. wheat germ

Combine all ingredients and blend until the consistency is of coarse cornmeal. Store and refrigerate in an air-tight container. When ready to use, combine 3 cups of mix with ¾ cup water (or milk) and shape into ball. Roll out on a floured board and cut into biscuits. Bake at 425° for 10 to 12 minutes.

Nutritional information per biscuit   164 calories, 4 g protein, 20 g carbohydrate, 8 g total fat, 2 g saturated fat, 3 g monounsaturated fat, 3 g polyunsaturated fat, .4 mg cholesterol, 2 g dietary fiber, 225 mg sodium

Applesauce Raisin Muffins

12 muffins

○ ☆ ⊠ ▨ *Healthy muffins have replaced donuts for breakfast. The applesauce in these muffins keeps them moist and delicious. A wonderful idea for brunch or a snack anytime. This recipe is another nutrition all-star.*

1½ cup uncooked oats
1¼ cup flour
¾ tsp. cinnamon
¼ tsp. nutmeg
1 tsp. baking powder
¾ tsp. baking soda
1 cup unsweetened applesauce
½ cup lowfat milk
½ cup firmly packed brown sugar
3 tbs. vegetable oil
1 egg white
½ cup raisins

Topping

1 tbs. brown sugar
¼ tsp. cinnamon
⅛ tsp. nutmeg
1 tbs. melted margarine

Combine all muffin ingredients. Fill greased muffin tins to ¾ full. Combine topping ingredients and sprinkle over muffin batter. Bake at 400° for 20 minutes or until golden brown. Serve warm or freeze for later use.

Nutritional information per muffin 198 calories, 4 g protein, 34 g carbohydrate, 5 g total fat, 1 g saturated fat, 2 g monounsaturated fat, 3 g polyunsaturated fat, 1 mg cholesterol, 2 g dietary fiber, 105 mg sodium

Popovers

4 large popovers

Popovers make a nice change for breakfast and they're delicious to serve with fruit, especially if you have children visiting. How many children ever heard of a popover? Reduce the fat to 10 grams for each popover by using only 2 eggs and cutting the margarine back to 2 tablespoons.

3 eggs
1 cup lowfat milk
3 tbs. melted margarine
1 cup flour
½ tsp. salt

Beat eggs until frothy. Mix in milk and melted margarine. Slowly beat in flour and salt. Batter should be light but not foamy. (Strain batter if it becomes lumpy.) Generously grease custard cups or popover pan. Fill each cup to within ½" of top. Bake at 400° for 45 to 50 minutes. Cut slits to allow steam to escape when done. Let stand in oven for 5 minutes.

Nutritional information per popover 276 calories, 10 g protein, 27 g carbohydrate, 14 g total fat, 4 g saturated fat, 6 g monounsaturated fat, 4 g polyunsaturated fat, 161 mg cholesterol, 1 g dietary fiber, 448 mg sodium

Raspberry Coffee Cake

Servings: 12

We chose this because it is similar to the texture of a sour cream coffee cake but made with lowfat yogurt. It is moist and delicious, and fresh raspberries make any dish special.

2 cups flour
1 tsp. baking powder
3/4 tsp. baking soda
1/4 tsp. cinnamon
1/4 tsp. nutmeg
1 1/4 cup fresh rasp-
  berries

1/2 cup margarine
1/2 cup sugar
2 eggs
1/4 cup plain lowfat
  yogurt
2 tsp. vanilla

Topping

1 tbs. margarine
2 1/2 tbs. chopped pecans

2 tbs. sugar
1/2 tsp. cinnamon

Grease an 8"x8" square pan. Combine flour, baking powder, baking soda, cinnamon and nutmeg. In a separate bowl, toss raspberries with 1 tbs. flour mixture. Cream margarine and sugar; add egg and blend well. Combine flour and margarine mixtures. Add yogurt and vanilla; blend in raspberries. Pour into a prepared pan. Combine topping ingredients; sprinkle over batter. Bake at 350° for 45 minutes or until cake tests done. Cool before serving.

Nutritional information per serving 225 calories, 4 g protein, 29 g carbohydrate, 10 g total fat, 2 g saturated fat, 5 g monounsaturated fat, 3 g polyunsaturated fat, 35 mg cholesterol, 1.5 g dietary fiber, 194 mg sodium

Strawberry Bread

Servings: 12

We took an old favorite recipe and lightened it by using unsweetened strawberries (fresh or frozen both do well) and less sugar. Whole wheat flour added wholesome whole grain and fiber. Remember how we used to bake in those 1-pound coffee cans for a different shape? Just the right size for gifts—a friend would love a loaf.

> 1½ cups whole wheat flour
> ½ tsp. baking soda
> ½ cup sugar
> 2 eggs
> ½ cup vegetable oil
> 2 tsp. orange peel
> ½ tsp. almond extract
> 2 cups chopped, unsweetened strawberries

Combine dry ingredients. In a separate bowl, lightly beat eggs. Add oil, orange peel and almond extract to eggs. Stir both mixtures together; fold in strawberries. Pour batter into 2 greased 1-pound coffee cans or 2 mini-loaf pans (3"x6"). Bake at 350° for 1 hour or until bread tests done. Let bread cool 10 minutes before removing from cans.

Nutritional information per serving   184 calories, 3 g protein, 21 g carbohydrate, 10 g total fat, 1 g saturated fat, 3 g monounsaturated fat, 6 g polyunsaturated fat, 35 mg cholesterol, 3 g dietary fiber, 46 mg sodium

Banana Bread

Servings: 12

◐ ☆ ⊠ ▨ *This nutrition all-star has a very pleasing flavor because of the lemon and honey. It's low in fat, cholesterol and sodium and provides a good source of fiber. Bake in 1-pound coffee cans, cool, pop the plastic top back on and store in your freezer. Or bake in mini-loaf pans.*

1 cup whole wheat flour
½ tsp. baking soda
¼ cup vegetable oil
¼ cup honey
1 egg, beaten
½ tbs. lemon peel
1 cup mashed banana

In a large bowl, combine dry ingredients. In a separate bowl, combine remaining ingredients. Stir both mixtures together. Pour batter into 2 greased 1-pound coffee cans or 2 greased mini-loaf pans (3"x6"). Bake at 350° for 45 minutes or until bread tests done. Let bread cool 10 minutes before removing from cans.

Nutritional information per serving 118 calories, 2 g protein, 17 g carbohydrate, 5 g total fat, 1 g saturated fat, 1 g monounsaturated fat, 3 g polyunsaturated fat, 17 mg cholesterol, 2 g dietary fiber, 63 mg sodium

No-Oil Spice Bread

Bread is the staff of life and this nutrition all-star proves it. A foolproof recipe, it is packed full of complex carbohydrates and fiber with only 1 gram of fat per serving. The gentle spice flavor is great with fruit.

2 cups whole wheat flour
¾ cup brown sugar
1 tbs. baking powder
1 tsp. baking soda
1 tsp. allspice
1 tsp. cinnamon
1 cup buttermilk
1 egg
¼ cup honey

Combine all ingredients. Pour mixture into a greased 9"x5"x2" loaf pan and bake at 350° for 50 minutes or until bread tests done.

Nutritional information per serving   94 calories, 2 g protein, 21 g carbohydrate, 1 g total fat, .2 g saturated fat, .2 g monounsaturated fat, .2 g polyunsaturated fat, 11 mg cholesterol, 2 g dietary fiber, 111 mg sodium

Wheat Germ Bread

Servings: 20

🦷 ⭐ 🌾 *This delicious, quick bread is eggless and oil-free. A slice contains only 1 gram of fat. Keep it low in fat by using a fruit spread instead of butter or margarine. Whole wheat flour and wheat germ need to be kept in the refrigerator or freezer to stay fresh.*

2½ cups whole wheat flour
1½ cups wheat germ
⅓ cup brown sugar
½ tsp. salt
1 cup raisins
2 tsp. baking soda
1¾ cups buttermilk
⅓ cup molasses

Combine flour, wheat germ, brown sugar, salt and raisins in a large bowl. Combine soda, buttermilk and molasses in a separate bowl. When the buttermilk mixture begins to bubble, stir in dry ingredients. Pour stiff dough into a greased 9"x5"x2" loaf pan. Bake at 350° for 1 hour or until bread turns light brown.

Nutritional information per serving 126 calories, 4 g protein, 27 g carbohydrate, 1 g total fat, .3 g saturated fat, .2 g monounsaturated fat, .5 g polyunsaturated fat, .8 mg cholesterol, 3 g dietary fiber, 162 mg sodium

Swedish Oven Pancake

Try this for breakfast when you have a house guest. We chose it because one serving has considerably less cholesterol than an egg. For a change, instead of sugar and lemon juice, use a fruit spread.

> 1½ tsp. margarine
> 2 eggs
> 1 cup lowfat milk
> 1 tsp. sugar
> ½ tsp. salt
> ½ cup *plus* 2 tbs. flour
> 2 tsp. confectioner's sugar (optional)
> 2 tsp. lemon juice (optional)

Melt margarine in oven in 9"x9" pan or pie plate. Beat eggs well. Add milk, melted margarine from pan, sugar, salt and flour. Pour batter into hot pan and bake at 400° for 15 to 20 minutes until pancake is puffy and lightly browned. Cut into 4 portions and serve hot. Sprinkle with confectioner's sugar and lemon juice if desired.

Nutritional information per serving   159 calories, 7 g protein, 20 g carbohydrate, 5 g total fat, 2 g saturated fat, 2 g monounsaturated fat, 1 g polyunsaturated fat, 109 mg cholesterol, 1 g dietary fiber, 348 mg sodium

5. Soups

How to Prepare and Freeze Homemade Broths

Servings: 6

⬭ ✦ ✉ *Are you tired of salty bouillon cubes or the high-sodium content of many canned soups? Do you long for the richness of homemade stock? It's not very difficult to make your own by simmering a chicken or meat bones with vegetables and seasonings. Use it in place of canned chicken broth or bouillon cubes in soups and other recipes.*

Basic Beef or Chicken Broth

6 cups cold water
2-3 lbs. chicken parts or 2-3 lbs. beef
   bones
1 onion, chopped
2-3 carrots, chopped
2-3 stalks celery, chopped
1 bay leaf
pepper, parsley and thyme to taste

Combine ingredients in a large pot and simmer for about 1 to 2 hours. Strain, chill and skim off fat. Stock may be stored in the refrigerator for several days or in the freezer for up to 6 months. If you freeze your stock in ice cube trays and store the frozen cubes in freezer bags, you'll always have homemade broth available in small amounts.

Nutritional information per 1-cup serving 12 calories, .1 g protein, 2 g carbohydrate, .5 g total fat, .2 g saturated fat, .3 g monounsaturated fat, .1 g polyunsaturated fat, 2 mg cholesterol, .3 g dietary fiber, 5 mg sodium

Mom's Potato Soup

Servings: 5

Homemade broth gives this soup its rich, but not salty, flavor. It also reduces the sodium to one third of the original recipe. You can reduce the sodium even further to 67 milligrams by eliminating the salt and adding herb mix or additional chopped fresh parsley. Thinning with lowfat milk adds a calcium boost to the lowfat high carbohydrate potato.

3 medium potatoes, peeled and sliced
1 medium onion, chopped
1 cup chopped celery
1 tbs. margarine
2 cups **Basic Chicken Broth,** page 46
1 bay leaf
1/4 tsp. salt
1 cup lowfat milk
1/8 tsp. paprika
1 tbs. chopped fresh parsley

In a heavy pot, sauté potatoes, onion and celery in margarine. Add chicken broth to cover potatoes. Add bay leaf. Simmer vegetables until tender, about 15 minutes. Remove bay leaf and add salt. Blend mixture in a blender or food processor until smooth. Add milk, heat and garnish with parsley and paprika.

Nutritional information per 1-cup serving   128 calories, 3 g protein, 21 g carbohydrate, 3 g total fat, 1 g saturated fat, 1 g monounsaturated fat, 1 g polyunsaturated fat, 5 mg cholesterol, 2 g dietary fiber, 186 mg sodium

Easy Gazpacho

This is a great chilled soup for summer. Make it ahead of time and store it in the refrigerator. It has nearly as much vitamin C as a glass of orange juice and provides almost 100% of the day's requirement for this vitamin. It's also a good source of vitamin A, especially beta-carotene. The original recipe called for whole milk, but we substituted lowfat milk. Result? It looks and tastes like a cream soup, but only has 3 grams of fat per serving.

1 (10¾ oz.) can condensed tomato soup
1 tsp. oregano
1 cup lowfat milk
½ cup chopped cucumber
¼ cup chopped green onion
¼ cup chopped green pepper
¼ cup croutons

Combine soup, oregano and milk. Chill until ready to serve. When serving, pour into bowls and sprinkle remaining ingredients over soup.

Nutritional information per ½-cup serving 98 calories, 4 g protein, 16 g carbohydrate, 3 g total fat, 1 g saturated fat, 1 g monounsaturated fat, 1 g polyunsaturated fat, 5 mg cholesterol, 1 g dietary fiber, 586 mg sodium

Five Ways to Make Cream Soup

Soup is a quick and delicious addition to any meal. Use this lowfat "cream" soup base and add your favorite vegetables.

Cream Soup Base

Servings: 4

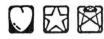

2 tbs. margarine
¼ cup chopped green onions
2 tbs. flour
1½ cups homemade chicken broth
1½ cups lowfat milk
½ tsp. salt (omit if using canned broth or bouillon cubes)
⅛ tsp. pepper

Melt margarine and sauté onion. Add flour and cook until bubbly. Add broth and blend well. Add remaining ingredients and cook over medium heat until mixture thickens, stirring constantly. Simmer 5 minutes.

Nutritional information per ¾-cup serving   90 calories, 4 g protein, 9 g carbohydrate, 5 g total fat, 2 g saturated fat, 2 g monounsaturated fat, 1 g polyunsaturated fat, 8 mg cholesterol, 0 g dietary fiber, 85 mg sodium

Try the following variations or create one of your own. There is only ¹⁄₁₀ of the sodium as compared to canned soups, plus you get the calcium boost from the lowfat milk and a chance to use healthy vegetables. Don't stay away from these "cream" soups—they are lowfat and don't have one speck of cream in them.

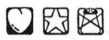 **Cream of Corn Soup.** Cut corn from three ears and add to soup base. Add 2 tbs. chopped green pepper. Simmer on low heat 10 minutes.

Nutritional information per 1-cup serving 154 calories, 6 g protein, 24 g carbohydrate, 5 g total fat, 1.5 g saturated fat, 1.5 g monounsaturated fat, 1.5 g polyunsaturated fat, 8 mg cholesterol, 3 g dietary fiber, 95 mg sodium

Cream of Broccoli Soup. Cook 1½ cups coarsely chopped broccoli until tender. Add to soup base and simmer 5 minutes.

Nutritional information per 1-cup serving 109 calories, 5 g protein, 12 g carbohydrate, 5 g total fat, 2 g saturated fat, 2 g monounsaturated fat, 1 g polyunsaturated fat, 8 mg cholesterol, 2 g dietary fiber, 90 mg sodium

Cream of Spinach Soup. Thaw ½ of a (10 oz.) package of chopped spinach and drain excess liquid. Add to soup base with dash of nutmeg. Simmer 10 minutes.

Nutritional information per 1-cup serving 100 calories, 5 g protein, 11 g carbohydrate, 5 g total fat, 2 g saturated fat, 2 g monounsaturated fat, 1 g polyunsaturated fat, 8 mg cholesterol, 1 g dietary fiber, 115 mg sodium

Cream of Chicken Soup. Steam ½ cup cut celery until tender. Add celery, 1 cup chopped cooked chicken and 1 tbs. chopped pimiento to soup base. Simmer 10 minutes.

Nutritional information per 1-cup serving 155 calories, 13 g protein, 10 g carbohydrate, 7 g total fat, 2 g saturated fat, 2 g monounsaturated fat, 2 g polyunsaturated fat, 37 mg cholesterol, 1 g dietary fiber, 121 mg sodium

Easy Carrot Bisque. Add 1 (4½ oz.) jar *each* strained baby food squash, carrots and applesauce to soup base. Add ⅛ tsp. curry powder. Serve hot or cold, sprinkled with nutmeg.

Nutritional information per 1-cup serving 134 calories, 4 g protein, 19 g carbohydrate, 5 g total fat, 2 g saturated fat, 2 g monounsaturated fat, 1 g polyunsaturated fat, 8 mg cholesterol, 1 g dietary fiber, 97 mg sodium

Cucumber Soup

This soup will keep for several days in your refrigerator. It makes a great light lunch when garnished with fresh mint or sprinkled with chopped parsley and served with a salad. It also makes a delicious first course at dinner. We reduced the fat from 16 grams to 1 gram and the calories from 194 to 72 per serving by substituting nonfat yogurt for sour cream. If you use homemade chicken broth, you can reduce the sodium from 369 mg to 105 mg. Feel like experimenting? Add 1 cup chopped cooked spinach to the cucumber mixture when you blend the ingredients.

3 cucumbers, peeled and sliced
½ cup chopped onions
1 clove garlic, minced
2 cups canned chicken broth
2 cups nonfat yogurt
⅛ tsp. salt
⅛ tsp. white pepper
fresh mint or chopped chives (optional)

Place cucumber, onion, garlic and broth in a blender or food processor and blend thoroughly. Pour mixture in bowls and stir in remaining ingredients. Garnish with fresh mint or chopped chives, if desired. Serve chilled.

Nutritional information per 1-cup serving 72 calories, 5.6 g protein, 12 g carbohydrate, 1 g total fat, .2 g saturated fat, .1 g monounsaturated fat, .1 g polyunsaturated fat, 1.7 mg cholesterol, 2 g dietary fiber, 369 mg sodium

Fish Chowder

Here is a good choice for a winter meal. Serve with a good French bread or bread sticks. One serving provides ¼ the daily requirement for calcium, so important for bone strength. We used lowfat milk to reduce fat and calories. You can reduce it even further by eliminating the margarine, which we've added for flavor.

> ¾ lb. white fish fillets
> 1 cup water
> 2 slices bacon, cut into small pieces
> 6 potatoes, peeled and cubed
> 3 tbs. chopped onion
> 2½ cups lowfat milk
> 1 tbs. margarine
> ⅛ tsp. salt
> ⅛ tsp. paprika

Place fish in a saucepan, cover with 1 cup water and simmer 10 minutes. In a separate saucepan, fry bacon pieces until lightly brown. Add potatoes and onion to bacon and stir until onion is translucent. Add ½ cup water to potato mixture, cover and cook 10 minutes. Break fish into small pieces and add to potato mixture. Simmer 10 to 15 minutes. Add milk and bring to a boil. Stir in margarine, salt and paprika.

Nutritional information per 1-cup serving 366 calories, 25 g protein, 48 g carbohydrate, 8 g total fat, 3 g saturated fat, 3 g monounsaturated fat, 1 g polyunsaturated fat, 53 mg cholesterol, 3 g dietary fiber, 283 mg sodium

5. Salads

All-Purpose Herb Mix

Want to add taste without adding calories or salt? Just mix these herbs and spices together and put them in a shaker. Add a few kernels of uncooked rice to prevent caking. Sprinkle on your favorite foods during cooking or at the table.

2 tsp. onion powder
1 tsp. garlic powder
1 tsp. paprika
1/2 tsp. thyme
1/8 tsp. white pepper
1/8 tsp. celery seed
1/8 tsp. sage
1 tsp. dried parsley

Tantalize your tastebuds!

- Add herb mix to soups and stews.

- Add herb mix to bread crumbs or cracker crumbs to make seasoned crumbs.

- Add herb mix to flour for seasoned breading for roasts or chicken.

Use herb mix along with these other herbs:

- tarragon for chicken dishes

- basil or oregano for tomato or Italian dishes

- rosemary for beef and lamb

- fresh parsley for any meat, fish, poultry or vegetables

- dill for potato salad, green beans and fish

Herbs and Spices: Use Your Imagination

Herbs and spices are used to enhance, not over-power, the flavor of foods. They are popular in cooking because they add so much flavor without using salt and fat.

- Dried herbs lose their flavor over a period of time. Check color for indication of strength; the darker or brighter the color, the more pungent and sharper the flavor. Revive dried herbs by soaking in lemon juice for several hours.

- Use about ¼ tsp. dried herbs or 1 tsp. fresh herbs per pound of meat, per pint of sauce or for every 4 servings of food.

- Dried herbs and spices retain their flavor best if pulverized just before using. Try rubbing them between the palms of your hands.

- Many fresh herbs can be frozen. Chop, label and freeze.

- If a recipe calls for a ground herb or spice and all you have is fresh or dried, remember: ⅓ tsp. powdered = 1 tsp. crushed = 1 tbs. fresh.

- Herbed butters are made from 1 tbs. fresh herbs to 1 stick butter or margarine. This mixture can be frozen in small dollops for later use.

- Chop fresh herbs finely or mash them with a mortar and pestle to release their oils. Sautéing herbs in oil or margarine helps draw out their flavor.

- Herbed vinegars are made from ½ cup fresh herbs to 1 pint vinegar. Basil, tarragon and garlic go well in white vinegar; oregano, rosemary, thyme, basil or marjoram in red wine vinegar. Heat vinegar to simmering and pour into a clean jar over the herb. Cool, cover and let steep 48 hours. Strain, if desired, and add a fresh herb for eye appeal. Herbed vinegars make great gifts!

- Add ½ cup fresh basil or tarragon to your favorite vinaigrette dressing.

- Jazz up salads by tossing in mint, dill, chervil or watercress with salad greens.

- By all means, grow fresh herbs beside your back steps, in a corner of your garden, or in pots on the windowsill in your kitchen. You'll find it's easy to do, and you'll really love the flavor of freshly picked herbs!

Salad Nicoise

Servings: 4

This adaptation of the classic French salad is easy to prepare and especially popular for luncheons. It is a good source of niacin and provides half the daily requirement for selenium and vitamin C. We cut back on olives in the original recipe and used water-packed tuna to reduce the fat. Then we changed to low calorie Italian salad dressing, and nobody could tell the difference! We reduced the fat by 16 grams and saved 144 calories. You can reduce the cholesterol to 23 milligrams if you use only the white part of the hard-cooked egg. One large egg has over 200 milligrams of cholesterol, and it's all in the yolk.

½ lb. fresh or 1 (10 oz.) pkg. frozen green beans
2 medium new potatoes, cooked, sliced
½ cup chopped green or mild onion
1 (6½ oz.) can water-packed tuna
10 ripe olives, sliced
2 tbs. chopped pimientos
1 hard-cooked egg, sliced
1 tbs. drained capers
½ cup low calorie Italian salad dressing
1 tomato, cut in wedges
lettuce leaves (as needed)

Blanch green beans until tender-crisp. Combine beans, potatoes, onion, tuna, olives, pimiento, egg and capers. Lightly toss with dressing. Serve on lettuce leaves, garnished with tomato wedges.

Nutritional information per serving 206 calories, 17 g protein, 27 g carbohydrate, 6 g total fat, 1 g saturated fat, 3 g monounsaturated fat, 1 g polyunsaturated fat, 76 mg cholesterol, 5 g dietary fiber, 451 mg sodium

Steak Salad

This is the perfect meal-in-one salad. Add bread and dessert and you are ready for guests! For those with heartier appetites, start with soup. We made our old recipe lower in fat and cholesterol by cutting down on oil and hard-cooked eggs. We tossed the ingredients together so that everything was lightly coated, rather than swimming in oil, and found that it tasted fresher and better that way. We also used olive oil, high in monounsaturated fatty acids, which are considered important in controlling cholesterol in the body.

2 tbs. olive oil
2 tsp. white wine vinegar
2 tsp. lemon juice
2 tsp. tarragon
1/8 tsp. dry mustard
1/2 head leaf lettuce, torn into pieces
1 lb. cooked steak, cubed
4 new potatoes, cooked and cubed
1 hard-cooked egg, sliced
6 cherry tomatoes
1 red onion, thinly sliced
1/2 cup sliced mushrooms
2 tbs. capers
2 tsp. prepared horseradish

Combine first 5 ingredients to prepare dressing. Set aside. Combine remaining ingredients. Add dressing to steak mixture and toss lightly to coat.

Nutritional information per serving 261 calories, 20 g protein, 22 g carbohydrate, 10 g total fat, 3 g saturated fat, 6 g monounsaturated fat, 1 g polyunsaturated fat, 81 mg cholesterol, 3 g dietary fiber, 120 mg sodium

Dilled Shrimp Salad

Make a day ahead for guests and serve on lettuce with tomato wedges and cold asparagus spears. We reduced the fat in the original recipe by decreasing the amount of sour cream and using light mayonnaise. We know that sour cream has a high percentage of fat and must be used in moderation, but it has ½ the fat of heavy cream and ⅕ the fat of butter for equal amounts. You can further decrease both fat and calories by using light sour cream. This recipe is high in cholesterol because of the shrimp, so you may want to watch the cholesterol in the other foods you eat during the day. Shrimp is low in fat and calories and an excellent source of iodine, part of the hormone secreted by the thyroid gland. Iodized salt is your best source of iodine, but if you've given up salt you may have to look to seafood.

> ¼ cup sour cream
> ¼ cup light mayonnaise
> 2 tsp. dill weed
> 1 lb. cooked shrimp, shelled
>   and deveined
> 1 cup seedless grapes
> 1 cup thinly sliced celery
> ¼ tsp. salt

Combine sour cream, mayonnaise and dill weed. Toss mixture with remaining ingredients. Refrigerate until ready to serve.

Nutritional information per serving 213 calories, 25 g protein, 11 g carbohydrate, 7 g total fat, 3 g saturated fat, 2 g monounsaturated fat, 2 g polyunsaturated fat, 232 mg cholesterol, 1 g dietary fiber, 498 mg sodium

Pasta Salad

Servings: 4

Many pasta salads are oily, but this one is a nutrition all-star. Pasta is high in complex carbohydrates and the fresh garden vegetables boost the vitamin content. This salad is a good way to use leftover macaroni or other cooked pasta. Be adventuresome! Try whole wheat pasta to boost fiber.

1 cup chopped tomatoes
½ green pepper, chopped
1 tbs. vegetable oil
6 oz. pasta, uncooked
¼ cup chopped green onion
1 tbs. oregano
2 tbs. olive oil
¼ cup sliced black olives
¾ cup uncooked frozen peas, thawed
¼ tsp. garlic powder
¼ tsp. salt
¼ tsp. pepper

Sauté tomatoes and green pepper in oil until slightly tender. Cook pasta according to package directions. Add pasta to tomato mixture. Add remaining ingredients and toss. Refrigerate until ready to serve.

Nutritional information per serving 97 calories, 2 g protein, 9 g carbohydrate, 7 g total fat, 1 g saturated fat, 4 g monounsaturated fat, 2 g polyunsaturated fat, 0 mg cholesterol, 2 g dietary fiber, 129 mg sodium

Shrimp and Pasta Salad

Servings: 4

Full of pasta for stamina and energy, this quick and easy salad is low in fat because we used less mayonnaise and more vegetables. It is high in selenium and also a good source of iron and calcium as well as vitamin C. If you don't have shrimp, try white chunk tuna packed in water. The broccoli alone in this recipe will supply almost all of the vitamin K you need for the day.

2 cups cooked pasta
1 cup cooked shrimp
1/4 cup chopped onion
1/2 cup chopped celery
1/4 cup sliced green onion
1 tbs. pimiento
1/2 cup light mayonnaise
1 cup chopped raw broccoli
1/4 cup pickle relish
1 tsp. celery seed
1 tbs. parsley
1/2 tsp. thyme
1/2 tsp. Worcestershire sauce
1/2 tsp. hot pepper sauce
1/4 tsp. salt
1/8 tsp. cayenne pepper (optional)

Combine all ingredients. Cover and chill until ready to serve.

Nutritional information per serving 245 calories, 16 g protein, 29 g carbohydrate, 7 g total fat, 1 g saturated fat, 2 g monounsaturated fat, 4 g polyunsaturated fat, 116 mg cholesterol, 3 g dietary fiber, 541 mg sodium

Curried Chicken Salad

Servings: 4

We included this recipe not only because of its healthy ingredients, but because it's one of our all-time favorites for entertaining, especially if you are serving a buffet. We think it tastes better if prepared a day in advance, and that will leave you free the day of your party. Serve with tomato wedges, chutney and fresh fruit kabob on bamboo sticks for a light and different taste. We lightened up our recipe by using lowfat milk and light mayonnaise. You could further lighten up by using a reduced-calorie creamy French dressing.

1½ cups cooked, chilled rice
1½ cups raw cauliflower pieces
¼ cup creamy-style French dressing
¼ cup light mayonnaise
1 tsp. curry powder
¼ tsp. pepper
2 tbs. lowfat milk
1⅓ cups (1 whole breast) chicken,
   cut into large chunks
⅓ cup sliced green pepper
½ cup chopped celery
⅓ cup thinly sliced red onion
½ tsp. salt

In a large bowl, combine all ingredients. Mix well. Cover and refrigerate until serving.

Nutritional information per serving 294 calories, 16 g protein, 26 g carbohydrate, 13 g total fat, 2.5 g saturated fat, 5 g monounsaturated fat, 5.5 g polyunsaturated fat, 41 mg cholesterol, 2 g dietary fiber, 580 mg sodium

Oriental Chicken Salad

This recipe is a delightful change of pace for chicken salad. We lightened it up by reducing the sesame oil from 3 to 2 tablespoons and by using a low sodium soy sauce (available in most grocery stores next to the regular variety). These small changes eliminated 4 grams of fat, 36 calories and 320 milligrams of sodium. The Chinese cabbage is a good source of vitamin A, especially beta-carotene, and also adds vitamin C, vitamin K and folate.

> 1½ cups cooked chicken
> 1/2 head Chinese cabbage
>   (approximately 3 cups)
> 2 tbs. low sodium soy sauce
> 3 tbs. sugar
> 2 tbs. sesame oil
> ½ tsp. grated fresh ginger
> ⅛ tsp. white pepper

Cut chicken into strips and set aside. Core cabbage, wash and cut into strips. Blanch, covered, in a microwave on high for 3 minutes or in boiling water or a steamer for 2 minutes. Drain. Combine soy sauce, sugar, oil, ginger and pepper in a saucepan. Bring to a boil; boil for several minutes. Combine chicken with cabbage and pour hot sauce over top. Serve hot or cold.

Nutritional information per serving   180 calories, 15 g protein, 11 g carbohydrate, 8 g total fat, 1 g saturated fat, 3 g monounsaturated fat, 4 g polyunsaturated fat, 36 mg cholesterol, 1 g dietary fiber, 228 mg sodium

Our Favorite Chicken Salad

Servings: 4

This chicken salad can be made a day ahead. We used light mayonnaise to cut down on fat and calories. Light mayonnaise has ½ the calories of the regular variety. Even though coconut is high in saturated fat, the amount of saturated fat in this recipe is balanced by the other fat sources (chicken, almonds, light mayonnaise) which are very low in saturated fat. This is an example of our philosophy that there is no good or bad food—it's how you use it and how much you use that makes the difference. This salad is also a great source of niacin.

1½ cups (1 whole breast) cooked diced chicken
1½ cups seedless green grape halves
4 oz. drained pineapple chunks
½ cup light mayonnaise
½ cup chopped celery
½ cup sliced water chestnuts
¼ cup slivered, toasted almonds
2 tsp. lemon juice
1 tsp. soy sauce
½ tsp. curry powder
⅛ tsp. Worcestershire sauce
½ cup shredded coconut

Combine all ingredients except coconut. Cover and chill for 2 hours. When ready to serve, sprinkle coconut over salad.

Nutritional information per serving 319 calories, 16 g protein, 29 g carbohydrate, 16 g total fat, 6 g saturated fat, 5 g monounsaturated fat, 5 g polyunsaturated fat, 44 mg cholesterol, 4 g dietary fiber, 316 mg sodium

Five Ways to Lightly Dress Your Salad

- Drizzle dressing lightly over your salad, rather than placing a 500-calorie (½ cup) mound of dressing on its center. Or better still, toss your salad with a very small amount of dressing in a large bowl before putting it on a serving plate. It doesn't take much dressing to coat the ingredients this way!

- Be skimpy with mayonnaise and oil in salad recipes (try 1:1 vinegar and oil and you'll grow to like it better), or make dressings with a "lite" mayonnaise or oil-free mix.

- Try balsamic vinegar or a rice wine vinegar on your salad. Many Europeans eat their salads this way without adding oil.

- Try sprinkling herbs and a little lemon juice on salad greens in place of a creamy or oily dressing.

- Experiment with reduced calorie or oil-free salad dressings.

Party Lime Salad

Horseradish is the ingredient that makes this salad special. We used lowfat cottage cheese and light mayonnaise to cut back on fat. You can save 50 calories per serving by using low calorie gelatin and you won't be able to tell the difference. You can further reduce the fat content with light sour cream or lowfat yogurt instead of regular sour cream.

½ cup boiling water
1 (3 oz.) pkg. lime gelatin
½ cup light mayonnaise
½ cup sour cream
½ cup lowfat cottage cheese
⅓ cup drained crushed pineapple
1 tbs. prepared horseradish
¼ cup chopped pecans
fresh parsley (optional)
maraschino cherry halves (optional)

Stir boiling water into gelatin until completely dissolved. Combine remaining ingredients and stir into gelatin mixture before it begins to set. Pour into individual molds or a 2-cup mold. Chill until set. Unmold and garnish with parsley or drained cherry halves, if desired.

Nutritional information per serving   198 calories, 16 g protein, 7 g carbohydrate, 11 g total fat, 4 g saturated fat, 4 g monounsaturated fat, 3 g polyunsaturated fat, 15 mg cholesterol, 2 g dietary fiber, 201 mg sodium

Marinated Vegetable Salad

Servings: 6

Store it in the refrigerator as a low calorie snack. It contains cruciferous vegetables (broccoli family) which may help in the prevention of certain types of cancer. An excellent source of beta-carotene, it supplies almost the entire daily requirement. Sodium can be reduced by substituting an herb mix for the salt. Did you know that salt is our most concentrated source of sodium? One teaspoon contains about 2000 milligrams, and the daily maximum should be 3000.

2 carrots, sliced
1 yellow squash, sliced
1 zucchini squash, sliced
½ cup fresh broccoli florets
½ cup cauliflower pieces
1 tsp. seasoned salt
¼ tsp. garlic powder
1 cup low-calorie Italian dressing
4 green onions, chopped
2 cups leaf lettuce, torn into pieces

In a microwave, cook vegetables in a covered dish until slightly tender. (If you do not have a microwave, blanch vegetables in a saucepan.) While vegetables are hot, sprinkle with seasoned salt, garlic powder and Italian dressing. Toss well, cover and refrigerate for at least 6 hours. Drain vegetables and toss with chopped onion and lettuce.

Nutritional information per serving   47 calories, 1 g protein, 7 g carbohydrate, 2 g total fat, .3 g saturated fat, .7 g monounsaturated fat, .7 g polyunsaturated fat, 0 mg cholesterol, 2 g dietary fiber, 685 mg sodium

Pea and Peanut Salad

Servings: 4

Here's "no-cooking home cooking" at its best. It's easy to keep a package of frozen peas in the freezer and a jar of peanuts in the pantry. Peas and peanuts are good sources of zinc, which is sometimes deficient in the diets of older adults. This salad is low in fat and light on salt but it does not store well; eat it soon after preparation.

1½ cups frozen, uncooked peas
2 tbs. chopped celery
½ tsp. Worcestershire sauce
1 tbs. minced onion
3 tbs. salted peanuts
1 tbs. light mayonnaise

Combine all ingredients.

Nutritional information per serving 93 calories, 5 g protein, 10 g carbohydrate, 4 g total fat, 1 g saturated fat, 2 g monounsaturated fat, 1 g polyunsaturated fat, 1 mg cholesterol, 3 g dietary fiber, 112 mg sodium

Spinach and Orange Salad

Servings: 4

○ ☆ 🌾 *Spinach salads are popular these days, but most of them are high in fat and loaded with bacon and bacon grease. The only fat in this colorful salad comes from the almonds, which are low in saturated fat. We chose this salad because it is a good source of several vitamins and fiber: at least 1/4 the daily requirement for vitamin A (mostly in beta-carotene), folate, vitamin C and vitamin E.*

        2 cups fresh spinach leaves
        1 cup drained mandarin orange slices
        1/2 cup sliced mushrooms
        1/3 cup no-oil vinaigrette dressing
        1/4 cup toasted sliced almonds

Toss spinach, oranges and mushrooms with dressing. Place salad in 4 individual serving bowls. Sprinkle almonds over salad before serving.

Nutritional information per serving   107 calories, 3 g protein, 14 g carbohydrate, 5 g total fat, 1 g saturated fat, 3 g monounsaturated fat, 1 g polyunsaturated fat, 0 mg cholesterol, 3 g dietary fiber, 183 mg sodium

New Potato Salad

Very different than standard potato salad, this is an unusual and delicious addition to a picnic or cold buffet. It contains 50% of the iron and vitamin C needed each day and is an excellent source of fiber because of the potatoes. You can lighten up by reducing the fat to 3 tablespoons of olive oil and cutting the olives in half, leaving just enough to give the salad some color. These small changes will eliminate 36 calories and 4 grams of fat per serving.

1 lb. small red new potatoes
1/4 cup olive oil
1/4 cup spicy mustard
3 tbs. lemon juice
2 tsp. prepared Italian seasonings
1/8 tsp. pepper
1 cup chopped celery
1 cup chopped green pepper
1/2 cup chopped green onion
20 black olives, sliced
2 tbs. chopped fresh parsley

Scrub potatoes, cut into quarters and cover with water. Cook until tender; drain and cool. Combine olive oil, mustard, lemon juice and seasonings. Add potatoes to oil mixture. Add remaining ingredients and toss. Chill until ready to serve.

Nutritional information per serving   185 calories, 3 g protein, 17 g carbohydrate, 13 g total fat, 2 g saturated fat, 9 g monounsaturated fat, 1 g polyunsaturated fat, 0 mg cholesterol, 4 g dietary fiber, 281 mg sodium

German Potato Salad

Servings: 4

This lowfat potato salad does not contain any mayonnaise. It only has 6 grams of fat, even with the bacon. Potatoes are a very good source of fiber and vitamin B6 as well as energy-boosting complex carbohydrates. You can lighten up even more by cutting back on bacon and omitting salt.

4 potatoes, peeled and sliced
3 strips bacon
1/2 cup chopped green onions
1/3 cup water
3 tbs. vinegar
1 tbs. sugar
1/4 tsp. salt
1/4 tsp. paprika
1/4 tsp. dry mustard
2 tbs. pimientos
2 tbs. chopped fresh parsley

Cook sliced potatoes in salted water until tender. Drain and set aside in a mixing bowl. Sauté bacon until crisp. Drain on paper towels. Pour off bacon fat except for 1 tbs. Sauté onions in bacon fat. In a saucepan, combine water, vinegar, sugar, salt, paprika and mustard; bring to a boil. Remove from heat; add onions and diced bacon to liquid mixture. Pour over potatoes, adding pimientos and parsley. Toss lightly.

Nutritional information per serving 194 calories, 4 g protein, 32 g carbohydrate, 6 g total fat, 2 g saturated fat, 3 g monounsaturated fat, 1 g polyunsaturated fat, 25 mg cholesterol, 2 g dietary fiber, 252 mg sodium

Freezer Coleslaw

Servings: 4

Here is an easy prepare-ahead slaw that keeps in the refrigerator for up to one week or can be frozen in single portions in freezer bags (can you believe that?). Cabbage is inexpensive, always available, and an excellent source (½ the daily requirement in one serving) of vitamin C. Cabbage is also an excellent source of vitamin K, important for blood clotting.

2½ cups shredded cabbage
2 tbs. grated carrot
2 tbs. chopped green pepper
2 tbs. chopped onion
¼ cup vinegar
1 tbs. water
½ cup sugar
¼ tsp. celery seed

Soak vegetables in salted water for 1 hour (add 1 tbs. salt to enough water to cover vegetables). In a saucepan, combine vinegar, water, sugar and celery seed to make dressing. Boil 1 minute and cool. Drain salt water from vegetables, add dressing and toss. Refrigerate several hours before serving.

Nutritional information per serving 112 calories, 1 g protein, 29 g carbohydrate, 0 g total fat, 0 g saturated fat, 0 g monounsaturated fat, 0 g polyunsaturated fat, 0 mg cholesterol, 1 g dietary fiber, 276 mg sodium

Artichoke and Asparagus Salad

Servings: 4

◌ ✪ ✉ 🌾 *This makes a good wintertime salad if fresh salad makings are scarce. It's packed with fiber and folate; most of its fat comes from olive oil, a monounsaturated fat which is recommended as a heart-healthy oil. You can use canned asparagus and artichoke hearts, but frozen vegetables contain less sodium than their canned counterparts.*

                1/4 cup lemon juice
                1/4 tsp. red pepper
                1 clove garlic, crushed
                1 tbs. olive oil
                8 artichoke hearts, frozen, cooked
                    or 1 (14 oz.) can unmarinated
                    artichoke hearts
                8 jumbo asparagus spears,
                    frozen, cooked
                4 red-tipped or leaf lettuce leaves
                1 tbs. sliced almonds
                6 ripe olives, sliced

Combine lemon juice, red pepper, garlic and olive oil. Pour mixture over artichoke hearts and asparagus spears; marinate at room temperature for 1 hour. Serve 2 artichoke hearts and 2 asparagas spears on a lettuce leaf, sprinkled with almonds and ripe olives.

Nutritional information per serving   95 calories, 3 g protein, 9 g carbohydrate, 6.5 g total fat, 1 g saturated fat, 4 g monounsaturated fat, 1 g polyunsaturated fat, 0 mg cholesterol, 6 g dietary fiber, 86 mg sodium

Tomato Salad Italian

When summer tomatoes are in season, this colorful and tasty salad offers a good source of vitamin C and fiber. The olive oil is a good choice because it is monounsaturated. You may think there is something special about the oil because it's cholesterol-free. But remember, cholesterol is only found in animal products, not fruits, vegetables, grains or vegetable oils.

    4 tomatoes, sliced
    1 small green pepper, sliced
    1 small Bermuda onion, sliced in rings
    ½ cucumber, sliced
    ½ cup wine vinegar
    ½ tsp. salt
    ½ tsp. pepper
    1 tsp. Italian seasoning
    1 tsp. chopped fresh parsley
    1 tbs. olive oil

Place sliced tomatoes, pepper, onion and cucumber in a bowl. Mix vinegar, pepper, Italian seasoning, parsley and olive oil in a measuring cup and pour over vegetables. Toss lightly and marinate at room temperature for 1 hour. Serve in salad bowls.

Nutritional information per serving 65 calories, 1 g protein, 9 g carbohydrate, 4 g total fat, 1 g saturated fat, 3 g monounsaturated fat, 0 g polyunsaturated fat, 0 mg cholesterol, 2 g dietary fiber, 276 mg sodium

Brown Rice Salad

Servings: 4

It's hard to come up with high fiber salads that are different from raw vegetables. Artichokes and brown rice are a great fiber combination and 6 grams of fiber is a lot, about ¼ of the daily recommendation. Using reduced calorie Italian dressing cuts calories and fat without sacrificing taste. This recipe is high in folate, too.

> 1 (14 oz.) can artichoke hearts, drained, unmarinated
> ¼ cup low calorie Italian dressing
> 1½ cups cooked brown rice
> ½ cup chopped green onions
> ¼ cup (8) sliced black olives
> ¼ tsp. curry powder
> 4 lettuce leaves

Cut artichoke hearts into quarters and marinate in Italian dressing for 4 hours. Mix rice, onions, olives and curry powder together. Combine with artichoke hearts and chill. Serve on lettuce leaves.

Nutritional information per serving   142 calories, 4 g protein, 26 g carbohydrate, 3 g total fat, .6 g saturated fat, 2 g monounsaturated fat, .7 g polyunsaturated fat, 0 mg cholesterol, 6 g dietary fiber, 221 mg sodium

7. Vegetables

Five Ways to Keep Your Vegetables Fresh

- Buy only what you will use. If a head of lettuce or other vegetable is going to spoil before you finish it, share it with a friend.

- If you use only small amounts of vegetables, consider buying just what you need from the supermarket salad bar. Some produce departments also package ready-to-use, cut-up vegetables in small portions.

- Tomatoes should be stored at room temperature until ripe, and then kept unwrapped in the refrigerator 2 to 3 days.

- If you wash your vegetables right after shopping, let them dry thoroughly before refrigerating to prevent rapid spoilage.

- Make soup with leftover vegetables. Soup can be stored for several days in the refrigerator and up to several months in the freezer.

Sweet Potato Casserole

Sweet potatoes are a favorite at holiday time. Because it is high in calories, save this casserole for a splurge, perhaps on your Thanksgiving or Christmas dinner menu. One serving provides all of the vitamin A needed in a day, mostly as beta-carotene. This old favorite, so popular in the South, called for 2 tablespoons of margarine. We eliminated that and reduced the fat by 5 grams per serving. You can further lighten up by skimping on the pecans, sugar and margarine—or just eat a smaller serving.

1½ cups cooked, mashed sweet potato
2 tbs. sugar
1 egg, beaten
½ tsp. vanilla
¼ cup lowfat milk

Topping

¼ cup light brown sugar
¼ cup flour
2 tbs. softened margarine
¼ cup chopped pecans

Combine sweet potato, sugar, egg, vanilla and milk. Pour into a 1-quart greased casserole dish. Combine topping ingredients until mixture is crumbly. Sprinkle topping over sweet potato casserole. Bake 25 minutes at 350°.

Nutritional information per serving 328 calories, 5 g protein, 50 g carbohydrate, 12 g total fat, 2 g saturated fat, 6 g monounsaturated fat, 3 g polyunsaturated fat, 53 mg cholesterol, 3 g dietary fiber, 169 mg sodium

Sweet Potatoes and Apples

Servings: 2

⬜ ⬜ ⬜ ⬜ *A nutrition all-star with all four symbols! This easy, colorful dish goes well with roasted turkey or a baked pork chop and gives you a daily supply of beta-carotene and vitamin A.*

> 1 sweet potato
> 1 apple
> pinch of cinnamon
> ⅛ tsp. lemon juice
> 1 tsp. margarine
> 1 tsp. brown sugar
> 2 tbs. water

Cook sweet potato until nearly done. Peel and slice potato into ½" round slices. Cut apple into wedges, leaving skin on. In a small, greased 1-quart baking dish, layer alternately 1 potato slice with 1 apple wedge. Sprinkle mixture with remaining ingredients. Bake covered at 350° for 15 minutes or until apple is soft.

Nutritional information per serving 125 calories, 1 g protein, 27 g carbohydrate, 2 g total fat, .4 g saturated fat, .9 g monounsaturated fat, .7 g polyunsaturated fat, 0 mg cholesterol, 3 g dietary fiber, 30 mg sodium

Oven-Baked Eggplant

Servings: 4

We chose this recipe because it was different from the standard preparations of this vegetable. A good source of fiber, eggplant soaks up oil like a sponge, so we avoided sautéing and baked it instead. Parmesan cheese is a whole milk cheese, but 3 tablespoons (1 oz.) goes a long way in adding flavor and calcium. You can lighten up this eggplant by cutting the mayonnaise in half.

1 small eggplant (about 1 lb.)
½ cup light mayonnaise
1 tbs. minced onion
¼ tsp. salt
⅓ cup Italian bread crumbs
⅓ cup Parmesan cheese

Wash eggplant. Peel and slice into ¾" slices. Set aside. Mix mayonnaise, onion and salt. Let stand 5 minutes. Brush both sides of sliced eggplant with mayonnaise mixture. Coat sliced eggplant with bread crumbs and Parmesan cheese. Place in a shallow pan coated with nonstick cooking spray. Bake at 425° for 15 to 17 minutes or until brown.

Nutritional information per serving   157 calories, 5 g protein, 16 g carbohydrate, 9 g total fat, 2 g saturated fat, 2 g monounsaturated fat, 3 g polyunsaturated fat, 14 mg cholesterol, 3 g dietary fiber, 472 mg sodium

Microwaved Acorn Squash

Servings: 4

⬜ ⬜ ⬜ ⬜ *Another nutrition all-star, this quick and easy recipe is low in fat, full of fiber and has little sodium. Winter squash has a sweeter taste than its summer cousin. You can cut down on calories by using apricot fruit spread instead of preserves. Fruit spreads are readily available in most supermarkets right beside the regular jams and jellies. They have about half the calories of their sweeter counterparts. We actually like the recipe better with fruit spread.*

> 1 acorn squash (approximately 1 lb.)
> ⅛ tsp. nutmeg
> dash of salt (optional)
> 2 tsp. margarine
> 2 tbs. apricot preserves
> 2 tbs. chopped pecans

Wash squash. Pierce with a knife in 2 places and place on a microwave-proof plate. Cook on high for 2 minutes. Cut squash into quarters lengthwise and remove seeds and fibers. Turn squash cut side up and sprinkle each piece with nutmeg and dash of salt, if desired. To each piece add ½ tsp. margarine, 1½ tsp. preserves and 1½ tsp. pecans. Cook covered on high for 4 minutes or until squash is tender. Remove cover and let stand for 5 minutes before serving.

Nutritional information per serving 133 calories, 2 g protein, 24 g carbohydrate, 4 g total fat, 1 g saturated fat, 2 g monounsaturated fat, 1 g polyunsaturated fat, 0 mg cholesterol, 3.5 g dietary fiber, 28 mg sodium

Baked Stuffed Acorn Squash

This recipe is great for fall holiday meals. It's low in fat and will contribute to the fiber and calcium in your diet. And it's delicious, too!

> 1 medium acorn squash
> 1 cup water
> 2/3 cup chopped onions
> 1 tbs. margarine
> 3/4 cup chopped fresh mushrooms
> 2 tsp. chopped fresh parsley
> salt and pepper (optional)
> 1/3 cup shredded cheddar cheese
> 1 tbs. bread crumbs

Cut squash into halves and scoop out seeds. Bake cut side down in a shallow pan with 1 cup water at 350° for 35 to 40 minutes. Sauté onions in margarine until tender. Add mushrooms and parsley and sauté briefly. Scoop squash out of shells and season with salt and pepper, if desired. Add onion, mushrooms and parsley; mix well. Cut shells in half and fill with mixture. Sprinkle cheese and bread crumbs on top of each shell. Return squash to oven until cheese melts.

Nutritional information per serving 110 calories, 4 g protein, 11 g carbohydrate, 6 g total fat, 3 g saturated fat, 2 g monounsaturated fat, 1 g polyunsaturated fat, 10 mg cholesterol, 2 g dietary fiber, 106 mg sodium

Potato Zucchini Casserole

Servings: 4

Potatoes, zucchini and part-skim mozzarella cheese are combined in a healthy and festive side-dish. It can be prepared a day ahead and reheated. (Use caution in freezing; potatoes do not freeze well for long periods of time.)

1 large potato
1 tbs. margarine
1 egg
2 oz. grated part-skim mozzarella cheese (½ cup)
¼ cup Parmesan cheese
1 small zucchini squash, grated
2 tbs. minced onion
¼ tsp. pepper
1 tbs. fresh minced parsley
1 tbs. dry bread crumbs

Boil potato. Drain, peel and mash in a large bowl. Add ½ tbs. margarine, egg, cheeses, zucchini, onion, pepper and parsley. Stir until well-combined. Sprinkle a greased 1-quart casserole with ½ tbs. bread crumbs. Spoon mixture into casserole and smooth top with spatula. Sprinkle remaining crumbs on top. Dot with remaining margarine. Bake at 400° for 20 minutes. Cut into 4 wedges or squares.

Nutritional information per serving 186 calories, 12 g protein, 12 g carbohydrate, 10 g total fat, 5 g saturated fat, 4 g monounsaturated fat, 1 g polyunsaturated fat, 72 mg cholesterol, 1 g dietary fiber, 291 mg sodium

Baked Potatoes Florentine

Servings: 4

Ⓞ ☆ 🌾 *Tired of the same old baked potato? Try
this one for a change. These potatoes
are attractive, different and nutritious, too. Potatoes
are a good source of complex carbohydrates and the
spinach is high in beta-carotene, supplying half of your
vitamin A for the day. Also a good source of vitamin C,
folate and fiber.*

2 large baking potatoes
1 cup chopped frozen spinach
2 tbs. margarine
2 slices bacon

Bake potatoes until tender. Cut in half lengthwise
after baking, scoop out potato and place pulp in a
mixing bowl. Cook spinach and drain excess liquid.
Add spinach and margarine to potato and mix until
well-blended. Spoon potato and spinach mixture
into potato skin shells. Cook bacon until crisp.
Crumble and sprinkle over stuffed potatoes. Bake
at 350° for 20 minutes.

Nutritional information per serving   192 calories, 5 g protein, 28 g
carbohydrate, 7 g total fat, 2 g saturated fat, 3 g monounsaturated fat, 2
g polyunsaturated fat, 3 mg cholesterol, 4 g dietary fiber, 166 mg sodium

Skinny Potatoes

◻ ◻ ◻ ◻ *These potatoes are crisp, brown and much lower in fat than French fries. And there's no mess or grease to clean up. Potatoes are good source of vitamin C and fiber.*

> 1 medium unpeeled baking potato (5"), sliced
> 1 tsp. vegetable oil
> ¼ tsp. paprika
> ¼ tsp. pepper
> ¼ tsp. garlic powder

Place potato slices on a cookie sheet. Baste with vegetable oil. Sprinkle with paprika, pepper and garlic powder. Broil for 5 minutes and turn. Broil until brown and crisp.

Nutritional information per serving 130 calories, 2 g protein, 26 g carbohydrate, 2 g total fat, .3 g saturated fat, .6 g monounsaturated fat, 1.4 g polyunsaturated fat, 0 mg cholesterol, 2 g dietary fiber, 8 mg sodium

Skillet Cabbage

◯ ⬚ ⬚ 🌾 *This nutrition all-star is low in fat, cholesterol and sodium. It's a good source of fiber, vitamin K and vitamin C. We chose this recipe since it is an easy way to dress up the humble cabbage, a member of the cruciferous vegetable family.*

2 tbs. margarine
2 tbs. chopped onion
2 tbs. chopped green pepper
4 cups shredded cabbage
1 tbs. flour
½ cup lowfat milk
¼ cup grated cheddar cheese
2 tbs. chopped pimiento

Melt margarine in a skillet. Sauté onion and green pepper for 5 minutes. Add cabbage, cover and cook for 10 to 15 minutes. Sprinkle flour evenly over cabbage. Gradually stir in milk. Cover and cook 3 to 5 minutes. Sprinkle with grated cheese and chopped pimiento.

Nutritional information per serving   121 calories, 4 g protein, 8 g carbohydrate, 9 g total fat, 3 g saturated fat, 3 g monounsaturated fat, 2 g polyunsaturated fat, 10 mg cholesterol, 2 g dietary fiber, 138 mg sodium

Nutty Broccoli

*Broccoli is one of the most popular cruciferous vegetables, a category we are encouraged to eat because of its possible protective role in cancer prevention. High in vitamins A, C and E, this recipe is also higher in fat than others. Our original recipe called for 1/2 cup of margarine and 3/4 cup of pecans, both concentrated sources of fat. By reducing these, we cut the fat from 25 grams to 14 and reduced the calories by 100. **Nutty Broccoli** has no cholesterol and lots of fiber, but remember to balance it with lowfat foods during the day.*

> 2 (10 oz. each) pkgs. frozen broccoli
>   florets or 3 cups fresh broccoli
> 1/4 cup margarine
> 1/2 pkg. dry onion soup mix
> 1/2 cup drained, chopped water chestnuts
> 1/2 cup chopped pecans

Heat frozen broccoli until it can be easily separated. If using fresh broccoli, steam 5 minutes. Place broccoli in a 1½-quart casserole dish. In a saucepan, melt margarine. Add soup mix, water chestnuts and pecans; mix well. Spoon mixture over broccoli. Bake at 350° for 10 to 15 minutes.

Nutritional information per serving   168 calories, 4 g protein, 9 g carbohydrate, 14 g total fat, 2 g saturated fat, 8 g monounsaturated fat, 4 g polyunsaturated fat, 0 mg cholesterol, 4 g dietary fiber, 165 mg sodium

Quick and Easy Stir-Fry

Stir-frying is a healthy way to cook vegetables. If you don't have a wok, a skillet works just as well. We used low sodium soy sauce to make our recipe healthier. Combine 3 or 4 of your favorite fresh vegetables. Good choices for stir-frying include broccoli, cauliflower, celery, green beans, onions, peppers, celery, mushrooms, pea pods, asparagus, zucchini and yellow squash. Stir-frying is a good way to use up small amounts of fresh vegetables in your refrigerator.

> 1 tbs. vegetable oil
> 1 clove garlic, minced
> 1/4 tsp. powdered ginger or 1 tbs. grated fresh ginger
> 1/2 lb. raw sliced vegetables
> 1 tsp. low sodium soy sauce

Heat oil. Add garlic and ginger; stir-fry 15 seconds. Remove garlic. Add vegetables and soy sauce. Stir-fry 3 to 5 minutes, stirring vegetables constantly until they become tender-crisp.

Nutritional information per serving 99 calories; 3 g protein, 7 g carbohydrate, 7 g total fat, 1 g saturated fat, 2 g monounsaturated fat, 4 g polyunsaturated fat, 0 mg cholesterol, 3 g dietary fiber, 84 mg sodium

Dilled Green Beans

Servings: 4

Use this quick and easy recipe for a cold vegetable or salad. It's particularly convenient if you are serving buffet-style because you don't have to worry about keeping it hot. We decreased the fat and calories by using light mayonnaise. You can decrease it further by using light sour cream instead of regular.

> 1 (9 oz.) pkg. frozen French-style
>   green beans
> 1/4 cup sour cream
> 1/4 cup light mayonnaise
> 1 tsp. dill weed
> 2 tbs. vinegar
> 1/4 cup chopped green onion
> 1/2 tsp. salt
> 2 tbs. chopped pimiento (optional)

Blanch beans for 1 minute and drain. Combine all ingredients. Refrigerate until cold.

Nutritional information per serving   86 calories, 1 g protein, 7 g carbohydrate, 6 g total fat, 2 g saturated fat, 2 g monounsaturated fat, 2 g polyunsaturated fat, 10 mg cholesterol, 2 g dietary fiber, 358 mg sodium

Microwaved Oriental Spinach

Servings: 4

⬭ ✦ 🌾 *This is a delightful change of flavor for spinach and a great accompaniment for pork, chicken, beef or lamb. Spinach is vitamin-packed (Popeye knew this!): one serving contains more than 50% of the beta-carotene needed every day, and it is also a good source of vitamin E, folate and fiber. You can lighten up by using low sodium soy sauce and reduce the sodium considerably.*

> 10 oz. fresh spinach leaves, torn
>   in pieces
> 8 oz. chopped water chestnuts
> 4 tbs. chopped green onion
> 1 tbs. vegetable oil
> 4 tbs. sweet and sour sauce
> 1 tbs. soy sauce

Place spinach in a 2-quart microwave-proof casserole dish. Add water chestnuts and onion. Microwave covered on high for 3 to 4 minutes or until spinach is limp. Stir, cover and set aside. Place oil and sauces in a 1-cup glass measure. Microwave on high for 1 minute. Pour sauce over spinach, toss and serve hot.

Nutritional information per serving 98 calories, 3 g protein, 15 g carbohydrate, 4 g total fat, 1 g saturated fat, 1 g monounsaturated fat, 2 g polyunsaturated fat, 0 mg cholesterol, 4 g dietary fiber, 624 mg sodium

Lentils and Brown Rice Casserole

Servings: 4

This meatless dish uses herbs and chicken broth to enhance its flavor. It's so easy—just throw all the ingredients together and bake! It freezes well (before cooking), too! High in fiber, folate and calcium, and low in fat and cholesterol. To lower sodium, use homemade chicken broth.

2 cups chicken broth
½ cup dry lentils
½ cup brown rice
¼ tsp. basil
⅛ tsp. thyme
1 garlic clove, minced
⅛ tsp. pepper
2 oz. part-skim mozzarella cheese, grated

Combine all ingredients, except ½ of the cheese. Pour mixture into a 1-quart ungreased casserole dish. Bake covered at 350° for 1 hour or until lentils and rice are tender. Uncover, top with remaining cheese and bake 2 to 3 minutes more.

Nutritional information per serving 208 calories, 12 g protein, 33 g carbohydrate, 3 g total fat, 2 g saturated fat, 1 g monounsaturated fat, 0 g polyunsaturated fat, 8 mg cholesterol, 4 g dietary fiber, 467 mg sodium

Vegetable Rice Supreme

To lighten up on sodium in this colorful dish, use homemade chicken broth or low sodium bouillon cubes. Rice is a good source of complex carbohydrate and the broccoli and tomatoes supply more than half of the vitamin C you need for the day.

 1/4 cup chopped onion
 3 tbs. margarine
 1 1/2 cups sliced mushrooms
 2 cups chopped broccoli
 1 cup chopped tomato
 2 cups water
 2 cubes chicken bouillon
 1 cup uncooked white rice
 1/2 tsp. oregano
 1/4 cup Parmesan cheese

Sauté onion in margarine until golden. Add mushrooms, broccoli and tomato. Cook until tender, approximately 4 minutes. Add water and bouillon cubes to mixture and bring to a boil. Stir in rice and oregano. Cover and cook over low heat about 20 minutes or until water is absorbed. Stir in Parmesan cheese. Serve hot or cold.

Nutritional information per serving 204 calories, 5 g protein, 30 g carbohydrate, 7 g total fat, 2 g saturated fat, 3 g monounsaturated fat, 2 g polyunsaturated fat, 3 mg cholesterol, 2 g dietary fiber, 514 mg sodium

Wild Rice Casserole

Servings: 4

A delicious complement to poultry or game, wild rice alone can be expensive. We've combined it with brown rice for that reason. This recipe is high in cholesterol because of the liver. But in one small chicken liver, you get almost twice as much B12 as you need for the day, all of the vitamin A and 3/4 of the folate, all vitamins sometimes low in the diets of older adults. So, should you refuse to eat this casserole? Almost everything you read says you shouldn't eat liver anymore. However, a little nutrition know-how can help you balance your foodstyle. Limit your daily intake of cholesterol to 300 milligrams per day, and you can have this casserole or other animal foods containing cholesterol.

        1/4 cup uncooked brown rice
        3/4 cup boiling water
        1/2 cup uncooked wild rice
        1/4 tsp. salt
        2 cups water
        1 cup chopped onion
        1/2 cup chopped celery
        1/2 cup chopped green pepper
        4 chicken livers, finely chopped
        2 tbs. margarine
        1 tbs. tomato puree
        1 tbs. chopped fresh parsley
        1 tbs. sherry
        1 clove garlic, minced
        1/8 tsp. *each* tarragon, basil and oregano

Combine brown rice with boiling water in a saucepan. Cover and simmer over low heat for 30 minutes. Combine wild rice, salt and water in another saucepan. Bring to a boil; boil for 35 to 40 minutes or until water is absorbed. Combine two rice mixtures. Sauté onion, celery, pepper and chicken livers in margarine for 5 minutes. Add to rice mixture with remaining ingredients. Pour into a small casserole dish and bake at 350° for 20 to 25 minutes.

Nutritional information per serving   174 calories, 8 g protein, 19 g carbohydrate, 7 g total fat, 2 g saturated fat, 3 g monounsaturated fat, 2 g polyunsaturated fat, 126 mg cholesterol, 2 g dietary fiber, 228 mg sodium

Spinach Lasagna

🌙 ⭐ 🌾 *We call this "lazy lasagna," because you don't have to cook the noodles. The microwave's time-saving steps help to create this excellent meatless main dish, with nearly a day's supply of vitamin A and beta-carotene and almost as much calcium as a glass of milk (253 milligrams per serving). And an excellent source of folate.*

> ½ tsp. margarine
> ½ cup chopped onion
> 1 clove garlic, minced
> 1 (16 oz.) can chopped tomatoes
> ½ tsp. oregano
> 1 tsp. basil
> 1 tsp. brown sugar
> ¼ cup tomato paste
> 1 tbs. Parmesan cheese
> 1 cup lowfat cottage cheese
> 1 (10 oz.) pkg. frozen spinach,
>   thawed and drained
> 3 uncooked lasagna noodles
> ¾ cup grated part-skim mozzarella
>   cheese

In a small glass bowl, microwave margarine until melted. Stir in onion and garlic. Cover bowl and microwave on medium high for 1 minute. Add undrained tomatoes, spices, brown sugar and tomato paste. Cover bowl with a paper towel and microwave on high for 10 minutes. Stir in Parmesan cheese and set aside. In a separate bowl, mix cottage cheese and spinach. Assemble lasagna in a 9"x5"x2" glass loaf pan beginning with ¼ cup sauce mixture; then a layer of uncooked noodles, broken into thirds; cheese/spinach mixture; ½ mozzarella cheese; and ½ sauce again. Repeat, ending with sauce. Top lasagna with remaining mozzarella cheese. Cover pan with plastic wrap and microwave on high for 6 minutes, and then on medium high for 15 minutes. Let stand for 15 minutes before serving.

Nutritional information per serving 202 calories, 16 g protein, 29 g carbohydrate, 4 g total fat, 2 g saturated fat, 1 g monounsaturated fat, 1 g polyunsaturated fat, 9 mg cholesterol, 5 g dietary fiber, 541 mg sodium

8. Beef

Steak and Veggies in Foil

Servings: 2

Recognize this one? It was popular back in the 50's and 60's when we were looking for a fuss-free mess-free way to cook (before the days of the microwave). This was probably one of the first ideas for meal-in-one dinners, too. Lost your recipe? We still have ours, and we've adjusted it for you into a two-portion size, using lean beef and eliminating the butter which was supposed to be dotted over the top. We used to bathe everything in butter! How times have changed! This recipe is a good source of zinc, selenium, iron, protein and niacin. One serving supplies more than enough vitamin A for the entire day, thanks to the carrots.

> 1/2 lb. lean beef round steak
> 1/2 packet onion soup mix
> 2 medium carrots
> 1 stalk celery
> 2 medium new potatoes

Place steak in center of a piece of heavy-duty aluminum foil. Sprinkle soup mix over top of meat. Cut up vegetables and place on top of meat. Close foil over meat and vegetables and set on a cookie sheet. Bake at 450° for 1 hour or until done. (If cooking on a grill, place foil directly on rack and grill until done.)

Nutritional information per serving 378 calories, 36 g protein, 36 g carbohydrate, 9 g total fat, 3 g saturated fat, 4 g monounsaturated fat, 1 g polyunsaturated fat, 93 mg cholesterol, 5 g dietary fiber, 277 mg sodium

Beef Cabbage Surprise

Servings: 4

Prepare this great one-dish meal in a hurry. One serving supplies 1/3 of the zinc, almost 1/2 of the folate and more than enough vitamin C and vitamin K for the day. It's a good source of niacin and calcium. An added bonus: not many recipes will provide 6 grams of fiber! We lightened this old favorite by reducing the amount of meat and eliminating margarine, unnecessary with nonstick cookware and the fat from the beef. You can reduce sodium by leaving the salt out and flavoring with favorite herbs.

    2 onions, chopped
    3/4 lb. lean hamburger
    1 (11 oz.) can tomatoes
    1 tsp. salt
    1/2 tsp. pepper
    1 medium head cabbage
    1 apple
    1/3 cup lemon juice
    1/4 cup sugar

Brown onion and hamburger in a nonstick Dutch oven or skillet. Stir in tomatoes, salt and pepper. Cover and cook for 20 minutes. Cut cabbage into coarse shreds; pare and chop apple. Stir cabbage, apple, lemon juice and sugar into mixture. Cover and cook another 30 minutes.

Nutritional information per serving 369 calories, 24 g protein, 34 g carbohydrate, 16 g total fat, 6 g saturated fat, 7 g monounsaturated fat, 1 g polyunsaturated fat, 74 mg cholesterol, 6 g dietary fiber, 782 mg sodium

Our Favorite Chili

This chili has real homemade flavor, and it freezes well, too. Package leftovers in small freezer bags for busy days. At 23 grams per serving, it's a concentrated source of protein because of the beef and beans. You only need 63 grams of protein per day if you're a man, and 50 grams if you're a woman. The recipe also supplies good amounts of niacin, zinc, iron and folate. The beans give you 9 grams of fiber per serving. Worried about the 16 grams of fat? It's almost all from the beef. Meat always has a higher percentage of fat than fruit, vegetables and grains. But don't eliminate it, because it contains many other nutrients that your body needs. Balance meats with lowfat foods during the meal or for the rest of the day.

    2 lbs. lean ground beef
    ½ cup chopped onion
    1 garlic clove, minced
    2 (15½ oz. each) cans dark red
        kidney beans
    2 (15½ oz. each) cans tomatoes
    1 (8 oz.) can tomato sauce
    1 pkg. chili sauce mix
    1 tsp. prepared horseradish
    1 tsp. hot sauce

Brown ground beef, onion and garlic. Add beans, tomatoes, tomato sauce and chili mix. Simmer 5 minutes. Add remaining ingredients. Simmer another 30 to 40 minutes.

Nutritional information per 1-cup serving 354 calories, 28 g protein, 24 g carbohydrate, 17 g total fat, 6 g saturated fat, 7 g monounsaturated fat, 1 g polyunsaturated fat, 74 mg cholesterol, 9 g dietary fiber, 797 mg sodium

Chinese Pepper Steak

Servings: 6

This dish looks lovely served over white rice, which is a good source of complex carbohydrate. Add a tossed salad or vegetable for a complete meal. One serving gives you almost a day's requirement for vitamin C and over half the requirement for vitamin B12. Also a good source of zinc and vitamin E, and only 204 calories. Who said we shouldn't include some beef in our diets? Just choose lean cuts and trim off all of the visible fat. By substituting low sodium soy sauce for the regular variety, we reduced the sodium from 770 milligrams per serving to 550 milligrams. You can eliminate more by using homemade or low sodium beef broth instead of a bouillon cube.

3 tbs. vegetable oil
1/2 tsp. salt
pepper to taste
1 lb. boneless sirloin steak
1/4 cup sliced onions
1 clove minced garlic
1 cup diagonally sliced celery
3 medium green peppers, sliced
1 beef bouillon cube
1 cup boiling water
2 tbs. cornstarch
1/4 cup water
2 tbs. low sodium soy sauce

Heat oil. Add salt and dash of pepper. Add sliced beef to oil and cook over high heat until beef is browned. Add onions and garlic and cook several more minutes. Stir in celery and green pepper. Cook, stirring constantly for 2 minutes more. Dissolve bouillon cubes in boiling water.

Add to meat mixture. Cover and cook over moderate heat until meat and vegetables are tender, about 20 minutes. Blend cornstarch into water and soy sauce. Add to meat mixture and stir until sauce thickens.

Nutritional information per serving 204 calories, 17 g protein, 6 g carbohydrate, 12 g total fat, 3 g saturated fat, 4 g monounsaturated fat, 4 g polyunsaturated fat, 43 mg cholesterol, 1 g dietary fiber, 550 mg sodium

Our Favorite Meat Loaf

Servings: 6

Meat loaf has come full circle since the 50's and is enjoying popularity even in restaurants! Use any that remains for sandwiches or pop it in the freezer for another meal.

1 lb. lean ground beef
1 cup (approximately 16) crushed saltine crackers
½ cup chopped onion
¼ cup chopped green pepper
½ cup chopped celery
1 egg, beaten
1 (8½ oz.) can stewed tomatoes
½ tsp. garlic powder
½ tsp. salt
¼ tsp. pepper

Combine all ingredients and mix lightly. Place in a 7"x3"x2" loaf pan or shape into a loaf and place in a baking dish. Bake at 325° for 1 to 1½ hours.

Nutritional information per serving 215 calories, 16 g protein, 9 g carbohydrate, 12 g total fat, 5 g saturated fat, 5 g monounsaturated fat, 1 g polyunsaturated fat, 87 mg cholesterol, 1 g dietary fiber, 410 g sodium

Beef Burgundy

You can make this company recipe days ahead and freeze it. All you have left to do is cook noodles or rice and make a salad. This recipe is packed with nutrition and only has 361 calories per serving. It contains ⅔ of the daily need for niacin, 60% of the vitamin E, and almost half of the zinc, iron, riboflavin and selenium.

2 lbs. top sirloin or round steak
3 tbs. vegetable oil
1 cup chopped onion
2 bay leaves
1 tsp. salt
¼ tsp. pepper
1 tsp. thyme
1 tsp. garlic powder
½ cup flour
2 cups red burgundy wine
¼ cup cognac (optional)
1 (10½ oz.) can beef broth
1 lb. fresh mushrooms, sliced

Cut steak into 1" cubes. Heat oil and sauté steak until brown. Place steak in a 2-quart baking dish with onions and bay leaves. Combine salt, pepper, thyme, garlic powder and flour. Stir dry mixture into burgundy, cognac (if used) and broth. Pour mixture over steak. Cover and bake at 325° for 1 hour. Add mushrooms and cook 30 minutes more or until steak is tender.

Nutritional information per serving 361 calories, 36 g protein, 14 g carbohydrate, 17 g total fat, 5 g saturated fat, 6 g monounsaturated fat, 5 g polyunsaturated fat, 87 mg cholesterol, 2 g dietary fiber, 597 mg sodium

Our Favorite Beef Brisket

Servings: 8

Best brisket in town! Serve as an entrée with vegetables or use for sandwiches. Be sure to trim all fat, or have the butcher do it for you. As people get older, they often have inadequate intakes of zinc, which is essential for many enzymes in the body. One serving of this recipe provides almost half the daily zinc requirement and is also a very good source of selenium and niacin. And more B12 than you need for the whole day.

2½ lbs. well-trimmed beef brisket
½ cup beef broth
3 oz. soy sauce
2 tbs. lemon juice
1 tsp. minced garlic
1½ tsp. liquid smoke
1½ tsp. Worcestershire sauce
½ cup barbecue sauce

Place brisket in a baking dish. Combine all ingredients except barbecue sauce and pour over brisket. Marinate 24 hours, turning beef only once. Bake covered at 300° for 3 hours or until done. Baste with barbecue sauce during last ½ hour.

Nutritional information per serving 204 calories, 32 g protein, 2 g carbohydrate, 7 g total fat, 3 g saturated fat, 3 g monounsaturated fat, .5 g polyunsaturated fat, 74 mg cholesterol, .1 g dietary fiber, 424 mg sodium

Chili Rarebit

Are you a grandparent? Children love this one and it's a nutrition powerhouse. Although higher in fat than many entrées because of the meat and cheese, a serving has 1/3 the adult daily requirement of niacin and zinc, almost half the iron, over half the protein and folate, and all the B12. It is also a good source of calcium, phosphorus and selenium. And it has 17 grams of fiber because of the beans. Balance the high fat content by serving over rice or on a bun along with a relish plate and fruit.

3/4 lb. lean ground beef
1 tsp. chili powder
2 (16 oz. each) cans kidney beans
1/2 cup shredded cheddar cheese
1/4 cup chopped onion

Brown ground beef in a nonstick skillet. Sprinkle with chili powder. Drain excess fat from skillet. Add 1 can drained and 1 can undrained kidney beans to beef. Stir constantly until heated thoroughly. Add cheese and stir until partially melted. Serve with chopped onion garnish.

Nutritional information per 1¼-cup serving   419 calories, 31 g protein, 35 g carbohydrate, 17 g total fat, 8 g saturated fat, 7 g monounsaturated fat, 1 g polyunsaturated fat, 70 mg cholesterol, 17 g dietary fiber, 929 mg sodium

French Bread Pizza

This easy pizza is better for you than take-out pizza and cheaper, too. Not only does it have as much calcium as a glass of milk because of the cheese, but it is also a good source of vitamin A. You can make it a complete meal by adding extra vegetable toppings such as mushrooms and green peppers.

1 small loaf French bread (5"x2"),
   halved
2 tsp. olive oil
¼ cup spaghetti sauce
1 tbs. Parmesan cheese
¼ cup sliced fresh mushrooms
¼ cup chopped green pepper
2 tbs. onions
2 tbs. grated carrots
½ cup cooked lean ground beef
2 oz. part-skim mozzarella cheese

Slice bread in half lengthwise. Baste loaf with olive oil. Place bread under broiler for 1 minute until brown. Spread spaghetti sauce on bread and top with Parmesan cheese, vegetables, beef and mozzarella cheese. Bake at 350° for 10 minutes or until cheese melts.

Nutritional information per serving 336 calories, 19 g protein, 26 g carbohydrate, 17 g total fat, 6 g saturated fat, 8 g monounsaturated fat, 2 g polyunsaturated fat, 40 mg cholesterol, 2 g dietary fiber, 559 mg sodium

Veal Scallopini Provençale

Servings: 4

Veal is an expensive but elegant change when you entertain. Add noodles and a salad and you're ready for company. This meal can be made ahead, frozen and heated prior to serving. One serving has almost 100% of the niacin needed for the day, at least 60% of the vitamin E, and 75% of the vitamin B12.

1 lb. veal scallops, about ¼" thick
½ tsp. salt
⅛ tsp. pepper
2 tbs. flour
2 tbs. vegetable oil
2 cups fresh sliced mushrooms
½ cup chopped onion
½ cup dry white wine
½ cup fresh chopped tomatoes
1 tsp. dried tarragon

Sprinkle veal with salt, pepper and flour. Sauté in oil over medium heat 2 to 3 minutes on each side. Remove veal to a warm platter. Add mushrooms and onions to pan and sauté until onions are slightly golden. Add wine, tomatoes and tarragon; simmer for 2 minutes longer. Return veal to pan and continue simmering for 5 minutes.

Nutritional information per serving 250 calories, 30 g protein, 7 g carbohydrate, 11 g total fat, 2 g saturated fat, 3 g monounsaturated fat, 5 g polyunsaturated fat, 117 mg cholesterol, 1 g dietary fiber, 343 mg sodium

9. Pork, Lamb and Game

Pork Tenderloin in Piquant Sauce

good!!

Servings: 4

Serve this quick and easy dish with seasoned rice or stir-fried vegetables. Pork is leaner than it used to be and doesn't have as much fat as you might think. Pork is also one of the best sources of thiamine; one serving of this recipe will provide half of your day's requirement of this vitamin. It is also a good source of niacin, phosphorus, selenium, iron and zinc.

 ¾ lb. pork tenderloin
 1 slice bacon
 1 onion, chopped
 1 tbs. margarine
 6 small sweet pickles, minced
 1 tsp. capers
 1 tbs. minced fresh parsley
 ¼ tsp. salt
 ⅛ tsp. pepper
 2 tbs. vinegar
 ½ cup tomato sauce

Place tenderloin on a rack in a roaster or in a baking dish. Arrange bacon on top and bake uncovered at 350° for 30 minutes. Sauté onion in margarine. Add pickles, capers, parsley, salt and pepper. Stir in vinegar and tomato sauce; cook for 10 minutes. Slice tenderloin. Pour sauce over tenderloin before serving.

Nutritional information per serving 255 calories, 22 g protein, 14 g carbohydrate, 13 g total fat, 3 g saturated fat, 5 g monounsaturated fat, 3 g polyunsaturated fat, 73 mg cholesterol, 2 g dietary fiber, 640 sodium

Baked Pork and Sweet Potatoes

Servings: 4

Tasty and easy to prepare, this recipe is also full of nutrition goodies. Look at the fiber, 5 grams, which comes mostly from potatoes and prunes. The vitamin A, most of which is in the form of beta-carotene from the sweet potatoes, is more than needed for the day. Because pork is so high in thiamine, you'll get almost half of your daily requirement, plus good amounts of riboflavin, niacin, vitamin E, vitamin C and selenium. And only 324 calories for meat and potato! Don't believe it when they say pork is bad for you!

4 boneless loin pork chops, 3 oz. each
2 sweet potatoes
2 tbs. lemon juice
4 slices pineapple, packed in juice
8 pitted dried prunes
8 whole cloves
½ cup pineapple juice

Brown pork chops in a skillet without fat; remove from heat. Peel sweet potatoes, cut in half lengthwise and rub with lemon juice. Place potatoes cut side down on each pork chop and top each with a pineapple slice. Insert cloves inside each pitted prune and place around pork chops. Pour pineapple juice over entire mixture and cover. Cook over low heat for 45 minutes.

Nutritional information per serving 324 calories, 20 g protein, 43 g carbohydrate, 8 g total fat, 3 g saturated fat, 4 g monounsaturated fat, 1 g polyunsaturated fat, 58 mg cholesterol, 5 g dietary fiber, 54 mg sodium

Braised Pork Cubes

While this recipe has no symbols, it is about as low in fat as it can be unless a nonstick pan is used to brown the pork instead of oil. Choose well trimmed pork loin or pork roast and serve over lowfat nutritious brown rice, knowing that the pork alone provides half of the thiamine and almost half of the selenium and vitamin E you need in a day, as well as 30% of the niacin. This is the kind of dietary trade-off we should make, balancing high fat and lowfat foods to attain the desired overall level of fat in the diet.

½ lb. boneless pork, trimmed and cubed
1 tbs. vinegar
½ tsp. paprika
1 tsp. cumin
1 tsp. turmeric
¼ tsp. salt

1 small clove garlic, minced
⅛ tsp. pepper
2 tsp. vegetable oil
¼ cup orange juice
3 tsp. water
1 tsp. flour

In a large bowl, mix pork cubes with vinegar, paprika, cumin, turmeric, salt, garlic and pepper. Marinate mixture for 1 hour in refrigerator. Remove pork from marinade and drain on a paper towel. (Do not discard marinade.) In a skillet, heat oil. Sauté pork until brown. Add orange juice, reserved marinade and 1 tsp. water; simmer covered for 15 minutes. Combine flour with 2 tsp. water and add to mixture. Stir until thickened, about 2 minutes.

Nutritional information per serving   278 calories, 28 g protein, 6 g carbohydrate, 15 g total fat, 4 g saturated fat, 6 g monounsaturated fat, 4 g polyunsaturated fat, 96 mg cholesterol, .4 g dietary fiber, 355 mg sodium

Broiled Ham and Cheese Sandwich

Servings: 4

A little different twist makes a plain ham and cheese sandwich special. Lean ham is lower in fat than it used to be, but like other processed meats, it's still high in sodium. We used to butter the bread, but now we're using a little spicy mustard to cut down on fat and calories. The cheese will give you 340 milligrams of calcium, more than a glass of milk.

        1 (8 oz.) loaf French bread
        2 tsp. spicy mustard
        4 oz. lean cooked ham, sliced
        1 green pepper, thinly sliced
        4 oz. Swiss cheese, sliced

Split bread lengthwise. Spread both sides of bread with mustard. Layer ham, green pepper and cheese over bread. Bake at 300° until cheese begins to melt, about 10 to 12 minutes.

Nutritional Information per serving 317 calories, 20 g protein, 31 g carbohydrate, 12 g total fat, 6 g saturated fat, 4 g monounsaturated fat, 1 g polyunsaturated fat, 41 mg cholesterol, 1 g dietary fiber, 866 mg sodium

Lamb Curry

Tired of beef, chicken and fish? Travel across the world and enjoy the flavors of Indian cuisine. Serve with rice and use chutney as a condiment. One serving will give you half the protein you need for the day and 75% of the B12. It is also a good source of iron, niacin, zinc and vitamin E.

1 lb. lamb shoulder, cut into ½" cubes
1 tbs. vegetable oil
3 tbs. chopped onion
1 tbs curry powder
1 tbs. flour
1 beef bouillon cube
1½ cups boiling water
¼ cup catsup
½ tsp. salt
½ cup chopped apple
1 cup diced celery

Brown lamb in oil over medium heat. Add onion and cook until translucent. Mix curry powder and flour, add to mixture and allow to bubble. Dissolve bouillon in boiling water and add to mixture. Add remaining ingredients and simmer for 1 hour.

Nutritional information per serving 317 calories, 31 g protein, 11 g carbohydrate, 16 g total fat, 6 g saturated fat, 6 g monounsaturated fat, 3 g polyunsaturated fat, 104 mg cholesterol, 2 g dietary fiber, 968 mg sodium

Cajun Duck

When all of the duck hunters bring home their game, here is an all-time favorite that has been served annually at game dinners. Its rich sauce makes a gravy even though wild duck is very low in fat. That's right, wild duck is not fatty like domestic duck, and a serving contains only 5 grams of fat. All of the vegetables in this recipe boost the fiber and vitamin C content, and **Cajun Duck** *is full of iron and niacin.*

4 wild duck breast halves
(about 1 lb.), deboned
⅛ tsp. black pepper
1 clove garlic, cut in half
1 clove garlic, minced
½ cup chili sauce
(tomato based)
½ cup chopped onion
½ cup chopped green
pepper
½ cup chopped celery
1 tsp. Worcestershire
sauce
1 tsp. dry mustard
1 tsp. nutmeg
2 tbs. lemon juice
½ cup water
¼ tsp. paprika
1 tbs. flour
1 tbs. water

Rub duck with pepper and garlic halves. Place duck in a baking dish and top with minced garlic. Combine chili sauce, onion, green pepper, celery, Worcestershire sauce, mustard, nutmeg, lemon juice and water. Pour over duck and bake at 325° for 1 hour. Mix paprika and flour with 1 tablespoon water and stir into sauce to thicken.

Nutritional information per serving   201 calories, 24 g protein, 14 g carbohydrates, 5 g total fat, 1.6 g saturated fat, 1.5 g monounsaturated fat, 1 g polyunsaturated fat, 82 mg cholesterol, 1 g dietary fiber, 547 mg sodium

Venison Goulash

This recipe was shared with us by a great hunter from the Alsace region of France. Beef can be substituted for venison if you don't have a deer hunter in the family. The combination of wine, spices and cream adds a gourmet flair. Venison is not very high in fat, so we splurged and used half and half in the recipe (our French hunter uses heavy cream). Don't forget, most of the calories in the wine disappear during cooking. All you need is noodles, a salad and some good French bread.

2 lb. venison, cut into 1" cubes	1 tsp. pepper
2 tbs. oil	½ tsp. cumin
2 small onions, sliced	½ tsp. coriander
1 garlic clove, minced	1 cup red wine
1 tbs. tomato paste	1 cup water
1 red bell pepper, chopped	1 cup half and half cream
3 tsp. paprika	1 tbs. dried oregano
	1 tbs. lemon juice

In a heavy skillet or Dutch oven, brown venison in oil. Lower heat and add onions, garlic, tomato paste and red bell pepper. Continue cooking for 1 minute. Stir in paprika, pepper, cumin, coriander, wine and water. Cover and simmer on top of stove or in a moderately low oven (325° for 1½ hours). Add more water if necessary to prevent sticking. Add cream, oregano and lemon juice; cook for 5 minutes.

Nutritional information per serving 312 calories, 37 g protein, 13 g carbohydrate, 12 g total fat, 5 g saturated fat, 3 g monounsaturated fat, 3 g polyunsaturated fat, 89 mg cholesterol, 3 g dietary fiber, 102 mg sodium

10. Chicken and Eggs

Five Easy Ways to Cook a Chicken Breast

Chicken breasts are the perfect quick food, especially if they are already deskinned and deboned, and even if they are still frozen when you begin to cook them. Most of the fat in chicken lies in the skin; remove it and reduce the fat by almost 50%. Here are quick-fix recipes. Remember, one chicken has two ½-breasts!

 Honey-Mustard Chicken   **Servings: 1**

> ½ chicken breast
> 1 tsp. honey
> 1 tsp. Dijon mustard
> dash curry powder and soy sauce
>   (optional)

Marinate chicken in honey, mustard and spices for several hours. Bake in aluminum foil or in a covered baking dish at 350° for 30 minutes or until done. (Note: Boneless breasts take only 15 minutes.)

Nutritional information per serving   166 calories, 27 g protein, 6 g carbohydrate, 3 g total fat, .8 g saturated fat, 1.3 g monounsaturated fat, .6 g polyunsaturated fat, 72 mg cholesterol, 0 g dietary fiber, 120 mg sodium

Easy Broiled Chicken   Servings: 1

½ chicken breast
2 tbs. low-calorie Italian dressing
2 tbs. tomato juice
dash chili powder or pepper sauce

Marinate chicken in mixture of dressing, tomato juice and spices for several hours. Broil or grill, basting frequently, until done.

Nutritional information per serving   162 calories, 27 g protein, 2.7 g carbohydrate, 4 g total fat, 1 g saturated fat, 1.5 g monounsaturated fat, 1 g polyunsaturated fat, 73 mg cholesterol, 0 g dietary fiber, 410 mg sodium

Italian Chicken   Servings: 1

½ boneless, skinless chicken breast
2 tbs. Italian bread crumbs
1 tsp. vegetable oil or margarine

Pound chicken to ½" thick. Roll in crumbs and sauté until done.

Nutritional information per serving   229 calories, 28 g protein, 9 g carbohydrate, 8 g total fat, 1.6 g saturated fat, 2.3 g monounsaturated fat, 3.4 g polyunsaturated fat, 73 mg cholesterol, .5 g dietary fiber, 155 mg sodium

Chicken Tarragon   **Servings: 1**

½ chicken breast
¼ cup white wine
1 tsp. dried tarragon leaves

Marinate chicken in wine and tarragon for several hours. Bake at 350° for 20 minutes or broil until tender.

Nutritional information per serving   180 calories, 26 g protein, 0 g carbohydrate, 3 g total fat, 1 g saturated fat, 1 g monounsaturated fat, .6 g polyunsaturated fat, 72 mg cholesterol, 0 g dietary fiber, 65 mg sodium

 Chicken Fajitas   **Servings: 1**

1 boneless, skinless chicken breast
2 drops soy sauce
1 tsp. lime juice
1 clove garlic, minced

Marinate chicken in soy sauce, lime juice and garlic. Grill or broil until done. Slice and roll up in a tortilla with your favorite Mexican filling such as sautéed onions, chopped tomatoes and a touch of sour cream.

Nutritional information per serving   147 calories, 28 g protein, 2 g carbohydrate, 3 g total fat, 1 g saturated fat, 1 g monounsaturated fat, 1 g polyunsaturated fat, 72 mg cholesterol, 0 g dietary fiber, 150 mg sodium

Baked Chicken in Pineapple

Servings: 4

Use this one for company when you know your guests are watching their calories: it's easy on the waistline. It's low in fat and high in fiber and will boost your iron intake for the day. Many people over 50 do not get enough vitamin C, B6 or B12. A serving of this recipe will supply almost 100% of your daily need for vitamin C and niacin and is also a very good source of B6 and B12.

2 whole chicken breasts, split in half
1/4 tsp. salt
1/8 tsp. pepper
1/2 tsp. curry powder
1 tbs. vegetable oil
1 onion, sliced
2 green peppers, sliced
1 cup crushed pineapple,
   packed in juice
1/3 cup brown sugar
1 (8 oz.) can sliced water chestnuts,
   drained
3/4 cup raisins

Sprinkle chicken with salt, pepper and curry powder. Heat oil in a skillet and brown chicken. Place browned chicken in a baking dish. Add remaining ingredients to skillet and cook over low heat for 15 minutes. Pour pineapple mixture over chicken and bake at 350° for 1 hour.

Nutritional information per serving 383 calories, 29 g protein, 57 g carbohydrate, 5 g total fat, 1 g saturated fat, 1 g monounsaturated fat, 3 g polyunsaturated fat, 68 mg cholesterol, 4 g dietary fiber, 226 mg sodium

Chicken and Capers in White Wine

So simple and so tasty! Capers will keep for a long time in your refrigerator and also can be used to jazz up other recipes. Low in fat, this has a day's worth of niacin.

4 tbs. flour
1 tsp. paprika
1/4 tsp. pepper
1/8 tsp. salt
1/2 tsp. garlic powder
1/2 lb. skinned chicken breasts
1/4 cup dry white wine
1/4 cup chicken broth
1 tsp. drained capers
1 tsp. chopped fresh parsley

Combine flour with seasonings. Dredge chicken in flour mixture. Place chicken in a small baking dish and pour wine and broth over it. Sprinkle with capers, cover with foil and bake at 450° for 15 minutes. Reduce heat to 325° degrees and continue baking until chicken is tender, about 15 minutes longer. (Cooking time will be reduced slightly if deboned chicken breasts are used in place of those with bones.) Sprinkle parsley over chicken just before serving.

Nutritional information per serving 199 calories, 29 g protein, 13 g carbohydrate, 3 g total fat, 1 g saturated fat, 1 g monounsaturated fat, 1 g polyunsaturated fat, 65 mg cholesterol, 1 g dietary fiber, 445 mg sodium

Company Chicken

Servings: 4

Another great entertaining recipe. Because you've removed the skin, you can use a little cream and still have only 9 grams of fat per serving. It's a good source of phosphorus, selenium, pantothentic acid, vitamin A and vitamin B6. Meat, fish and poultry are your most dependable sources of niacin and one serving will give you almost 100% of your daily requirement.

1 lb. chicken breasts, boneless
  and skinless
2 tbs. margarine
16 small white onions, peeled
1/2 tsp. salt
1/8 tsp. pepper
1/4 tsp. thyme
1 1/2 tsp. paprika
3/4 cup beer
1/4 cup tomato sauce
1 bay leaf
1/4 cup half and half

Brown chicken in margarine. Add onion and brown slightly. Add remaining ingredients, except half and half, and bring to a boil. Cover and simmer for 30 minutes. Stir in half and half.

Nutritional information per serving 273 calories, 29 g protein, 19 g carbohydrate, 9 g total fat, 3 g saturated fat, 3 g monounsaturated fat, 2 g polyunsaturated fat, 71 mg cholesterol, 3 g dietary fiber, 525 mg sodium

Mexican Chicken

This "south of the border" favorite uses tomato paste to give a boost in vitamin A. Although this recipe isn't as high in either fat or sodium as you might expect, you could reduce these nutrients by cutting the cheddar cheese back to ¾ cup without sacrificing any flavor. The secret is to use extra sharp cheddar to get the most flavor from the least amount of cheese.

1 (8 oz.) can tomato paste
1 pkg. chicken marinade mix or
  2 tsp. herbed chicken seasoning
½ tsp. chili powder
¼ tsp. ground cumin
½ cup chopped green onion
1½ lbs. skinless chicken breasts
¾ cup crushed tortilla chips
1 (2¼ oz.) can ripe olives,
  drained and sliced
1 cup shredded cheddar cheese

Thoroughly blend tomato paste, chicken marinade mix, chili powder, cumin and onions in a 9"x13" glass baking dish. Place chicken in marinade mixture. Turn. Pierce all chicken surfaces with a fork. Turn several more times and marinate 20 to 30 minutes. Bake uncovered at 400° for 30 minutes. Sprinkle with tortilla chips and olives. Top with cheese. Bake 10 minutes longer.

Nutritional information per serving 277 calories 33 g protein, 11 g carbohydrate, 11 g total fat, 5 g saturated fat, 4 g monounsaturated fat, 1 g polyunsaturated fat, 85 mg cholesterol, 3 g dietary fiber, 322 mg sodium

Chicken Artichoke Casserole

Servings: 4

It's hard to find recipes with this much fiber (7 grams), and it comes from the artichokes. Prepare in advance and heat just before serving. It's a good source of niacin, B12 and folate, and has as much calcium as a glass of milk. Lighten up on fat and sodium if you wish by cutting back on cheese to 1/2 cup.

2 whole chicken breasts (4 halves)
1 tbs. margarine
1/4 cup chopped green onions
1 clove garlic, minced
3 tbs. flour
2 cups lowfat milk
3/4 cup shredded cheddar cheese
1 cup sliced mushrooms
12 oz. artichoke hearts,
    drained and halved

Boil chicken until tender. Remove skin and bones and cut meat into large pieces. Set aside. Melt margarine and sauté onions and garlic. Add flour and stir fry until bubbly. Slowly add milk and cook over low heat until mixture thickens, stirring constantly. Add cheese and stir until melted. Stir in chicken, mushrooms and artichokes. Pour mixture into a casserole dish and bake at 350° for 20 to 30 minutes.

Nutritional information per serving 337 calories, 27 g protein, 20 g carbohydrate, 17 g total fat, 7 g saturated fat, 4 g monounsaturated fat, 5 g polyunsaturated fat, 67 mg cholesterol, 7 g dietary fiber, 277 mg sodium

Baked Eggs Florentine

Servings: 4

Great for brunch, one serving contains almost 100% of the daily vitamin A requirement and is a good source of beta-carotene because of the spinach. It also supplies ¼ of your calcium and ½ of your folate needs. Why so high in cholesterol? Because of the egg yolk. One egg has more than 200 milligrams cholesterol. But eggs are a good source of other nutrients and you shouldn't be afraid to use them in moderation. We recommend that you limit egg yolks to 4 a week, including those used in cooking.

1 (10 oz.) pkg. frozen chopped spinach
4 eggs
⅓ cup shredded cheddar cheese
1 cup condensed cream of celery soup

Cook spinach until just heated. Drain thoroughly, pressing all liquid from spinach. Press drained spinach into a well-greased 6"x6" casserole dish or individual ramekins.. With a large spoon, make an indentation in spinach for each egg. Carefully crack and drop an egg into each indentation. Sprinkle half of the cheese over casserole. Lightly beat soup and spread over egg and cheese mixture. Sprinkle casserole with remaining cheese. Bake at 325° for 20 to 25 minutes or until bubbly.

Nutritional information per serving   176 calories, 12 g protein, 9 g carbohydrate, 11 g total fat, 4 g saturated fat, 4 g monounsaturated fat, 2 g polyunsaturated fat, 225 mg cholesterol, 2 g dietary fiber, 660 mg sodium

Baked Eggs Supreme

Servings: 4

Although this recipe is a good source of both vitamin A and calcium, it is high in fat and cholesterol. That doesn't mean you have to give it up forever. Serve for a special brunch with fresh fruit and unbuttered muffins and watch the other foods you eat that day. Remember, it's the overall amount of fat and cholesterol you eat that is important, not what is in a single food.

4 oz. sliced fresh mushrooms
1 tbs. margarine
3/4 cup shredded Swiss cheese
1/4 cup lowfat milk
1/4 tsp. salt
1/8 tsp. pepper
1/2 tsp. dry mustard
4 eggs, slightly beaten
1 tbs. chopped parsley

Cook mushrooms in margarine until lightly browned and excess liquid evaporates from pan. Set aside. Sprinkle cheese in a well-greased 1-quart baking dish. Mix milk with salt, pepper and mustard. Pour half of mixture over cheese. Top with mushrooms and beaten eggs. Pour remaining milk mixture over all. Bake at 325° degrees for 30 minutes or until eggs are set. Sprinkle with chopped parsley.

Nutritional information per serving   195 calories, 14 g protein, 4 g carbohydrate, 14 g total fat, 6 g saturated fat, 5 g monounsaturated fat, 2 g polyunsaturated fat, 229 mg cholesterol, 1 g dietary fiber, 298 mg sodium

11. Fish

Easy Shrimp Creole

Servings: 6

The ingredients may sound unusual for a creole, but you'll be surprised and delighted. Serve over rice and be prepared to offer seconds on this one. Not only is this recipe easy to prepare, but it is also a good source of several nutrients which are not always easy to get. A serving will provide almost all the vitamin C you need for the day because of the tomato soup and green peppers. The evaporated milk, along with the shrimp, provide a good source of calcium. You'll also get iodine from the shrimp, and one serving will take care of 50% of your iron and 100% of your selenium needs for the day. You can lighten up by substituting evaporated skim milk and never know the difference.

2 tbs. vegetable oil
1 cup chopped green pepper
1 cup chopped onion
1 (10¾ oz.) can condensed tomato soup
1 cup evaporated milk
1 tbs. curry powder
¼ tsp. pepper
1½ lb. cooked shrimp, deveined

Heat oil in a large skillet. Add green pepper and onion; cook slowly until tender. Add soup, milk, curry powder and pepper. Simmer for 20 minutes, stirring occasionally. Add shrimp and cook over low heat for 10 minutes.

Nutritional information per serving 260 calories, 28 g protein, 14 g carbohydrate, 10 g total fat, 3 g saturated fat, 3 g monounsaturated fat, 4 g polyunsaturated fat, 233 mg cholesterol, 1 g dietary fiber, 653 mg sodium

Flounder Parmesan

Servings: 4

This is an old recipe which called for either sour cream or buttermilk. We chose buttermilk because with sour cream, the calories came to 251 and the fat was 14 grams. With buttermilk there are only 153 calories and 3 grams of fat. It also brought the cholesterol down a bit. Small change, big difference— but tastes just as good.

1 lb. flounder (other types of fish
  work well, too)
1 cup buttermilk
¼ cup Parmesan cheese
1 tsp. lemon juice
1 tbs. chopped onion
½ tsp. salt
⅛ tsp. hot pepper sauce
⅛ tsp. paprika
1 tbs. chopped fresh parsley

Place fish fillets in a well-greased 12"x8"x2" baking dish. Combine remaining ingredients, except paprika and parsley. Spread mixture over fish and sprinkle with paprika. Bake at 350° for 25 to 30 minutes or until fish flakes. Garnish with parsley.

Nutritional information per serving   153 calories, 26 g protein, 4 g carbohydrate, 3 g total fat, 2 g saturated fat, .8 g monounsaturated fat, .5 g polyunsaturated fat, 61 mg cholesterol, .1 g dietary fiber, 519 mg sodium

Poached Salmon
with Ginger Sauce

Servings: 4

Salmon is a heart-healthy food, and the sauce adds zest. Chinese stir-fried vegetables or sautéed snow peas are a good accompaniment. We reduced the sodium from 854 milligrams to 151 milligrams by substituting low sodium soy sauce for regular and by using homemade chicken broth. This dish will supply you with over half of the niacin and all of the B12 you'll need for the day.

3 cups home-made chicken broth
1 onion, sliced
2 tbs. vinegar
1 tsp. dill weed
1 bay leaf
1⁄8 tsp. pepper
4 salmon steaks (approx. 4 oz. each)

Heat chicken broth to boiling and add onion, vinegar, dill, bay leaf and pepper. Simmer 5 minutes. Add salmon, cover and steam for 8 to 10 minutes. Remove from pan and serve with ginger sauce.

Ginger Sauce

1 cup pineapple juice
1 tbs. vegetable oil
3 tbs. cornstarch
1 tbs. low sodium soy sauce
3 tbs. vinegar
½ cup water
½ cup sugar
2 tsp. grated fresh ginger (or 1 tsp.
   powdered ginger)

Cook pineapple juice and oil over low heat for several minutes. Add remaining ingredients and cook until thickened, stirring constantly. Serve over salmon steaks.

Nutritional information per serving   369 calories, 23 g protein, 44 g carbohydrate, 11 g total fat, 2 g saturated fat, 3 g monounsaturated fat, 5 g polyunsaturated fat, 63 mg cholesterol, 1 g dietary fiber, 155 mg sodium

Baked Fish Supreme

This is a terrific dish for the calorie-conscious. It only has 213 calories per serving and provides over 100% of the selenium and B12 you need for the day. Fish is one of the very best sources of B12, which is important in the formation of red blood cells, and is also important in the functioning of the central nervous system. Older adults often do not get enough B12.

2 tbs. margarine
1 tbs. chopped onion
½ cup chopped fresh mushrooms
½ cup dry white wine
1¼ lbs. white fish fillets
⅛ tsp. salt
⅛ tsp. pepper
3 tbs. bread crumbs
1 tbs. chopped fresh parsley

Heat margarine and sauté onion until translucent. Add mushrooms and sauté 1 minute more. Add wine and boil rapidly for 1 minute. Place fish in a shallow, greased baking dish and season with salt and pepper. Pour wine mixture over fish and sprinkle with bread crumbs. Bake at 425° for 15 to 20 minutes or until fish is just cooked and crumbs are golden and crisp. Garnish with parsley.

Nutritional information per serving 190 calories, 27 g protein, 2 g carbohydrate, 7 g total fat, 2 g saturated fat, 3 g monounsaturated fat, 2 g polyunsaturated fat, 68 mg cholesterol, .3 g dietary fiber, 260 mg sodium

Baked Fish Florentine

Servings: 4

Because of the spinach, this is an excellent source of beta-carotene and vitamin A. Beta-carotene has been associated with lower cancer risk and is found in dark green and deep yellow fruits and vegetables. **Baked Fish Florentine** *will also contribute to your calcium, folate, B12, selenium and phosphorus needs for the day. Delicious and low in calories too!*

1 lb. fish fillets
1 (10 oz.) pkg. frozen spinach souffle, thawed
8 Ritz round crackers, crushed
2 tbs. Parmesan cheese
lemon wedges for garnish

Place fish in a baking dish. Spoon spinach on top of fish. Combine crackers and Parmesan cheese and sprinkle over fish. Bake at 400° for 10 to 20 minutes or until fish flakes. Garnish with lemon wedges.

Nutritional information per serving   248 calories, 27 g protein, 6 g carbohydrate, 13 g total fat, 5 g saturated fat, 5 g monounsaturated fat, 2 g polyunsaturated fat, 147 mg cholesterol, 2 g dietary fiber, 566 mg sodium

Fuss-Free Fish Cooking

Bake: Place fish on a greased baking dish (or dish sprayed with nonstick cooking spray). Brush fillet with oil or a lowfat sauce and bake in a moderate oven (350°) until fish flakes.

Broil: Place fish on a greased broiler pan, about 4" from heat. Baste with oil or a lowfat sauce during broiling. Do not turn fish over unless it is very thick. Broil until fish flakes.

Poach: Fill a shallow frying pan with water seasoned with wine, vinegar, lemon juice, onion and bay leaf. Bring to a boil and add fish. Reduce heat and simmer until fish is done.

Oven Steam: Brush fish lightly with oil. Wrap tightly in heavy-duty aluminum foil. Bake at 450° degrees for 15 minutes for fish that is 1" thick. Add 5 minutes cooking time for each additional 1/2" thickness.

Microwave: Place fish in a microwave-proof dish and cover tightly with plastic wrap. Microwave on medium for 30 seconds. Turn dish and microwave another 30 seconds to 1 minute. Drain off juices and let stand covered for a few minutes before serving.

Shrimp in Wine

Servings: 6

Serve as a main dish or as a hot sandwich on toasted French rolls. It's low in calories and is a good source of selenium, vitamin A and iron. We lightened the original recipe by changing from 1 stick of butter to ½ stick of margarine, reducing fat from 16 to 9 grams per serving. This also saved 63 calories, enough to add an apple during the day.

¼ cup chopped green onion
1 tsp. minced garlic
¼ cup melted margarine
1½ lb. shrimp, peeled and deveined
1 tsp. lemon juice
¼ cup dry white wine
¼ tsp. salt
⅛ tsp. pepper
1 tsp. dill weed
1 tbs. chopped fresh parsley

Sauté onion and garlic in margarine until tender. Add shrimp, lemon juice, wine, salt and pepper. Cook over medium heat about 5 minutes, stirring occasionally. Add dill weed and parsley.

Nutritional information per serving   180 calories, 24 g protein, 1 g carbohydrate, 9 g total fat, 2 g saturated fat, 3 g monounsaturated fat, 3 g polyunsaturated fat, 221 mg cholesterol, .2 g dietary fiber, 431 mg sodium

Cheesy Salmon Patties

Servings: 4

You can turn a can of salmon into patties for an entrée and then eat the extras on buns with lettuce, tomato and light mayonnaise for lunch the next day. These patties contribute more than the daily requirement of selenium and vitamin B12 and are an excellent source of calcium. Be sure to mash up the bones in the salmon—that's where the calcium is and why canned salmon is such a good source of this important mineral.

1 (13 oz.) can boneless salmon
1 egg, beaten
½ cup seasoned bread crumbs
¼ cup shredded cheddar cheese
1 tsp. dried minced onion
1 tsp. garlic powder

Drain salmon, reserving 2 tbs. liquid. In a mixing bowl, combine all ingredients including the reserved liquid. Mix well and shape into 4 patties. Broil 5 minutes on each side until cheese is melted and patties are golden brown.

Nutritional information per serving 227 calories, 23 g protein, 10 g carbohydrate, 9 g total fat, 4 g saturated fat, 3 g monounsaturated fat, 2 g polyunsaturated fat, 107 mg cholesterol, .5 g dietary fiber, 663 mg sodium

Crab-Stuffed Eggplant

Servings: 4

Serve this high fiber entrée with a tossed salad and garlic bread for a complete meal. Shrimp can be substituted for crab meat.

2 small eggplants (1 lb. each)
1 onion, chopped
2 tbs. margarine
2 (4½ oz. each) cans crab meat
1 cup seasoned bread crumbs
1 egg, beaten
½ tsp. oregano
2 tbs. chopped fresh parsley
½ tsp. salt
⅛ tsp. pepper
2 drops hot pepper sauce

Slice eggplants in half lengthwise and parboil about 10 minutes. Remove from water, drain and scoop out centers. Place eggplant pulp in a mixing bowl and set aside. Slice eggplant shells in half lengthwise again, making 4 quarters. Sauté onion in margarine until tender. Add crab meat, ¾ cup bread crumbs and remaining ingredients to eggplant pulp. Mix well. Fill each shell with mixture and sprinkle with remaining bread crumbs. Place shells in a shallow baking dish with ¼ cup water poured into bottom. Bake at 350° for 30 to 35 minutes.

Nutritional information per serving 298 calories, 21 g protein, 32 g carbohydrate, 10 g total fat, 2 g saturated fat, 3 g monounsaturated fat, 5 g polyunsaturated fat, 110 mg cholesterol, 8 g dietary fiber, 688 mg sodium

Five Delicious Easy Ways to Cook a Fish Fillet

Get hooked on fish by trying these foolproof ways to cook a fish fillet. We all need to eat more fish and all of these ways are easy, tasty and still low in fat. When buying fish, make sure it is fresh. It should not have a strong fishy odor. Salt water fish contains iodine, an important mineral which is hard to get without iodized salt, which you are probably cutting down on.

 **Crispy Oven Fried Fish   Servings: 1**

½" thick fish fillet (4 oz. raw)
1 tsp. melted margarine
1 tbs. flour
¼ tsp. paprika
salt and pepper to taste (optional)

Place fish in a baking dish. Top with ingredients and broil 5 minutes.

Nutritional information per serving   162 calories, 22 g protein, 6 g carbohydrate, 5 g total fat, 1 g saturated fat, 2 g monounsaturated fat, 2 g polyunsaturated fat, 58 mg cholesterol, 0 g dietary fiber, 138 mg sodium

Fish with Tomato Cheese Topping

Servings: 1

½" thick fish fillet (4 oz. raw)
1 tsp. melted margarine
1 tsp. lemon juice
1 tbs. grated onion
½ cup fresh chopped tomato
1 tbs. shredded Swiss cheese
salt and pepper to taste (optional)

Place fish in a baking dish. Top with remaining ingredients except cheese and broil 5 minutes. When done, sprinkle with 1 tbs. shredded Swiss cheese and broil 1 minute longer.

Nutritional information per serving 181 calories, 24 g protein, 5 g carbohydrate, 7 g total fat, 2 g saturated fat, 2 g monounsaturated fat, 2 g polyunsaturated fat, 65 mg cholesterol, 2 g dietary fiber, 165 mg sodium

Broiled Fish with Herbs

Servings: 1

½" thick fish fillet (4 oz. raw)
1 tsp. melted margarine
1 tsp. chopped fresh parsley
1 tsp. chives
¼ tsp. tarragon
paprika, garlic powder, thyme, salt and pepper to taste (optional)

Place fish in a baking dish. Top with ingredients and broil 5 minutes.

Nutritional information per serving 133 calories, 21 g protein, 0 g carbohydrate, 5 g total fat, 1 g saturated fat, 2 g monounsaturated fat, 2 g polyunsaturated fat, 58 mg cholesterol, 0 g dietary fiber, 139 mg sodium

Barbecued Fish in Foil   Servings: 1

Good with fresh cod

½" thick fish fillet (4 oz. raw)
1 tbs. barbecue sauce

Place fish on a greased sheet of aluminum foil. Smear with sauce and bake at 350° for 15 minutes.

Nutritional information per serving   109 calories, 21 g protein, 2 g carbohydrate, 2 g total fat, .3 g saturated fat, .4 g monounsaturated fat, .4 g polyunsaturated fat, 58 mg cholesterol, 0 g dietary fiber, 216 mg sodium

 Grilled Salmon Fillet   Servings: 1

1 salmon fillet (4 oz. raw)
1 tsp. lemon juice
½ tsp. soy sauce

Marinate salmon in lemon juice and soy sauce for 1 hour. Grill or broil for 5 to 10 minutes.

Nutritional information per serving   186 calories, 23 g protein, 0 g carbohydrate, 9 g total fat, 2 g saturated fat, 5 g monounsaturated fat, 2 g polyunsaturated fat, 74 mg cholesterol, 0 g dietary fiber, 228 mg sodium

The secret to all great fish dishes is: don't overcook. Cooking fish too long makes it tough and destroys its delicate texture and flavor. Measure a fish fillet at its thickest part. For fresh, fully thawed fish that measures 1" thick, cook 10 minutes. Partially thawed (semi-frozen) fish should be cooked 12 to 15 minutes. Add 5 minutes for fish cooked in foil or in a sauce.

Paella

Excellent

Servings: 4

⬜ ⬜ 🌾 *This one-dish meal, adapted from a classic Spanish recipe, is nutrition-packed. Clams are a great source of iron. This recipe contains all of the iron and selenium needed in a day and half of the niacin. Selenium, a trace mineral, was recently added to the Recommended Dietary Allowances of foods needed by the body. Try variations with scallops, shrimp, fish, lean sausage or brown rice.*

w/mussels

4 oz. (1 cup) chopped
  raw chicken
1 tbs. olive oil
½ cup chopped onion
2 tomatoes, chopped
1½ cups homemade
  chicken broth
¾ cup uncooked white
  rice

1 tbs. paprika
¼ tsp. pepper
⅛ tsp. cayenne pepper
½ lb. fish fillets, cut in 1"
  pieces
1 can drained clams
½ cup frozen peas
2 tbs. pimientos,
  chopped

In a skillet, brown chicken in oil. Pat off excess oil and pour fat from pan. Add onion and tomatoes to slightly greased skillet and cook 5 minutes. Stir in broth, rice, paprika, pepper, and chicken. Simmer covered 20 minutes or until rice is almost done. Stir in fish, clams and peas and simmer 5 to 10 minutes longer. Add pimientos and heat thoroughly. (If using brown rice, parboil in chicken broth 30 minutes before adding onions, tomatoes, chicken and spices.)

Nutritional information per serving 328 calories, 29 g protein, 39 g carbohydrate, 6 g total fat, 1 g saturated fat, 3 g monounsaturated fat, 1 g polyunsaturated fat, 58 mg cholesterol, 3 g dietary fiber, 159 mg sodium

Spaghetti with Clam Sauce

Servings: 2

The *wonderful flavors of clams, Parmesan cheese and garlic make this a great pasta dish, and it's so easy. Most foods don't have much iron, but this dish is an outstanding source because of the clams. The original recipe called for a whole stick of butter, but we lightened up by reducing the fat by almost 90%. Add some shrimp or scallops to the recipe for a heartier entrée. The fresh parsley adds a wonderful taste.*

1 (6½ oz.) can clams
2 tsp. cornstarch
1 tbs. margarine
1 clove garlic, minced
1 tbs. chopped onion
¼ tsp. basil
1 tbs. chopped fresh parsley
1 tbs. Parmesan cheese
2 cups hot cooked spaghetti

Drain clams. Add water to clam juice to make 1 cup. Stir in cornstarch and set aside. Melt margarine in a skillet and sauté garlic, onion, basil and parsley. Add clam juice mixture and cook until thick, about 1 to 2 minutes. Stir in Parmesan cheese and clams and heat thoroughly. Pour over hot spaghetti.

Nutritional information per serving 335 calories, 20 g protein, 45 g carbohydrate, 8 g total fat, 2 g saturated fat, 3 g monounsaturated fat, 2 g polyunsaturated fat, 33 mg cholesterol, 2 g dietary fiber, 168 mg sodium

12. Desserts

Old-Fashioned Sugar Squares

40 squares

◻ ◻ ◻ *This is a simple and unusual version of sugar cookies. Our original recipe was titled **Grandma's Sugar Cookies** and had a note in a child's handwriting which simply said, "Yum!" This prudent delicious dessert or snack is not loaded with sugar or fat, and will be loved by everyone from 5 to 50+.*

1 cup margarine
1¼ cups sugar
2 eggs
2 cups flour
¼ tsp. baking soda
1 tsp. salt
1 tsp. powdered ginger
2 tbs. lowfat milk
½ tsp. lemon juice

Cream margarine and 1 cup of sugar. Add eggs and blend well. In a separate bowl, combine flour, baking soda, salt and ginger. In a small bowl, combine milk and lemon juice. Add flour mixture and liquids alternately to creamed mixture and blend. Spread batter evenly in a greased 15"x10"x1" pan. Sprinkle remaining sugar over top. Bake at 400° for 20 minutes. Cool and cut into squares.

Nutritional information per square   92 calories, 1 g protein, 11 g carbohydrate, 5 g total fat, 1 g saturated fat, 2 g monounsaturated fat, 2 g polyunsaturated fat, 10 mg cholesterol, .2 g dietary fiber, 116 mg sodium

Eggless Pumpkin Cake

Servings: 24

◩ ⬚ ⬚ ⬚ *There's no better way to get fiber than from this delicious pumpkin cake. One serving contains almost half of the vitamin A that you need for the day and a lot of vitamin E from the vegetable oil. And no eggs! Make 4 cakes and freeze 3 for later. Recipe can also be made into 1 bundt cake.*

    1 cup sugar
    ½ cup brown sugar
    1 cup vegetable oil
    1 (16 oz.) can pumpkin
    ⅔ cup water
    1 tsp. cinnamon
    ½ tsp. allspice
    3 cups whole wheat flour
    2 tsp. baking soda
    ½ tsp. salt

Combine all ingredients. Pour mixture into four 1-pound coffee cans, greased or sprayed with vegetable cooking spray. Bake at 350° for 45 minutes to 1 hour. Let cakes sit in coffee cans for 10 minutes; remove and cool on a rack.

Nutritional information per serving   186 calories, 2 g protein, 25 g carbohydrate, 9 g total fat, 1 g saturated fat, 2 g monounsaturated fat, 6 g polyunsaturated fat, 0 mg cholesterol, 2 g dietary fiber, 116 mg sodium

Summer Fruit Pie

Servings: 8

This naturally sweetened pie, with its bounty of summer fruits, contributes half of the daily requirement for vitamin C. The original recipe called for a homemade graham cracker crust, but a commercial graham cracker crust was used in the analysis, as you may choose it for convenience. The crust is high in fat so to lighten up, just use 3/4 cup of the crumbs on the bottom of the pie plate rather than the total crust. You can use any combination of fruits to change the color and flavor. Or try sponge-cake torte shells available in specialty food stores and some grocery stores for a good lowfat cake base.

> 9" graham-cracker crust or sponge-cake torte
> 2 sliced nectarines (or peaches)
> 1/2 cup blueberries
> 2 cups sliced strawberries
> 2 cups chunk pineapple
> 3/4 cup pineapple juice
> 2 tsp. cornstarch

Layer fruits on top of crust in pie pan. Save a few berries for garnishing. Blend pineapple juice with cornstarch in a saucepan and heat until thickened, stirring regularly. Pour thickened juice over fruit. Garnish with reserved berries. Refrigerate several hours until ready to serve.

Nutritional information per serving   271 calories, 3 g protein, 42 g carbohydrate, 11 g total fat, 2 g saturated fat, 5 g monounsaturated fat, 4 g polyunsaturated fat, 0 mg cholesterol, 3 g dietary fiber, 241 mg sodium

Five Ways to Serve Fresh Fruit

Fresh fruit has always been a popular food, even before the days of light meals and health-conscious dining. It can be used at any meal or for a snack. Fresh fruit is low in calories and contains little fat. Here's how to use fresh fruit to add elegance and taste to your meals:

- For a buffet luncheon or dinner, arrange strawberries, watermelon and cantaloupe cubes, maraschino cherries and canned pineapple cubes on bamboo skewers for a prepare-ahead, easy-to-serve salad kabob.

- Fruit and cheese make a great dessert or appetizer. Select your favorite cheese and add strawberries, grapes, melon, apple wedges or bing cherries. Arrange on a platter or on individual serving dishes. Garnish with parsley.

- Experiment with your favorite liqueurs. Sprinkle melon balls with a little lemon juice and add chopped fresh mint and cream de menthe. Add Grand Marnier and coconut to sliced oranges. Amaretto is delicious drizzled over raspberries or blueberries. Kirsch, cream de cassis, and many other liqueurs can enhance fresh fruits. For a special treat, serve fruit and liqueur over frozen yogurt or ice milk.

- Poach pears, apricots, peaches or nectarines and drizzle with your favorite liqueur or custard sauce (see *Cream Custard Sauce for Fruit,* page 151).

- Mix any orange-flavored liqueur with slightly softened orange sherbet and serve in hollowed-out orange halves. Add creme de menthe to lemon, lime or pineapple sherbet and serve in hollowed-out lemon shells. These desserts can be made the day before and frozen. Be sure to slice off a piece of rind from the bottom of the fruit shell so that it will sit upright on the plate. Garnish with fresh mint leaves or a maraschino cherry.

Cream Custard Sauce for Fruit

Servings: 4

Dress up your favorite fruit with this smooth-as-silk custard sauce that sounds rich, tastes rich but is low in fat. The evaporated skim milk boosts the calcium to 200 milligrams.

2 tbs. brown sugar
1 cup evaporated skim milk
1 egg, slightly beaten
½ tsp. vanilla
1 tbs. dark rum

Combine brown sugar and milk in a heavy saucepan. Cook over medium heat until mixture is hot. Gradually stir about ¼ of the hot mixture into the beaten egg; add remaining hot mixture, stirring constantly. Cook until mixture thickens, stirring constantly. Remove from heat and stir in vanilla and dark rum. Cover and chill. When ready to serve, stir custard with a wire whisk and spoon over fruit.

Nutrional information per 3-tbs. serving 102 calories, 6 g protein, 14 g carbohydrate, 1.4 g total fat, .5 g saturated fat, .5 g monounsaturated fat, .2 g polyunsaturated fat, 55 mg cholesterol, 0 g dietary fiber, 93 mg sodium

Amaretto Baked Apple

Servings: 1

⬭ ☆ ⬚ 🌾 *There is a great demand for low sugar desserts with a gourmet touch. The refreshing natural sweetness in the apple juice and the almond flavor in the amaretto liqueur are a unique combination. Add raisins, dates or ground almonds for a change. Apples are a good source of soluble fiber and an all-American favorite.*

> 1 tart baking apple
> 1 tbs. amaretto liqueur
> 1/8 tsp. cinnamon
> 1 tbs. apple juice concentrate
> 1/4 tsp. lemon juice
> 1 tbs. chopped almonds (optional)

Core apple to within 1" of bottom. Place apple in a small baking dish. Combine amaretto, cinnamon, apple juice and lemon juice; pour over apple. Bake uncovered in a 350° oven for 30 minutes. Sprinkle with chopped almonds, if desired.

Nutritional information per apple 110 calories, .4 g protein, 28 g carbohydrate, .5 g total fat, .1 g saturated fat, 0 g monounsaturated fat, .2 g polyunsaturated fat, 0 mg cholesterol, 4 g dietary fiber, 6 mg sodium

Blueberry Squares

Delicious served warm or cold. Use as a dessert, snack or bread. These squares freeze well for future use. Not as high in calories or fat as most desserts, they will still satisfy your sweet tooth.

> 2 cups flour
> 1 tbs. baking powder
> ¼ tsp. salt
> ⅓ cup margarine
> ¾ cup sugar
> 1 egg
> 1 tsp. vanilla extract
> ½ cup lowfat milk
> 2 cups fresh or frozen blueberries

Combine flour, baking powder and salt. Cream margarine with sugar, egg and vanilla until well-blended. Add milk and blend at low speed until just combined. Add flour mixture and blend one minute longer. Gently fold in blueberries. Bake in a greased 9"x9"x2" pan at 375° for 30 minutes or until golden brown. Let cool slightly before cutting.

Nutritional information per square 195 calories, 3 g protein, 32 g carbohydrate, 6 g total fat, 1 g saturated fat, 3 g monounsaturated fat, 2 g polyunsaturated fat, 18 mg cholesterol, 1 g dietary fiber, 198 mg sodium

Peach Cobbler

Quick, easy and delicious. You can use any seasonal fruit as a substitute for peaches. This is lighter than most desserts and a healthy way to add vitamins to your diet with fruit. The liqueur adds an interesting and subtle flavor, and the calories from the alcohol are mostly burned off during cooking.

- ¼ cup margarine
- ½ cup flour
- ½ cup sugar
- ½ tsp. baking powder
- ⅛ tsp. salt
- ¼ cup lowfat milk
- ¼ cup Grand Marnier, amaretto or kirsch
- 2 cups skinned, sliced peaches

Melt margarine in a 1-quart casserole. Mix together flour, sugar, baking powder and salt. Add milk and liqueur to flour mixture; beat until smooth. Pour into casserole. Place fruit on top of flour mixture. Do not stir. Bake at 350° for 40 minutes.

Nutritional information per serving   200 calories, 2 g protein, 31 g carbohydrate, 8 g total fat, 2 g saturated fat, 3 g monounsaturated fat, 2 g polyunsaturated fat, 1 mg cholesterol, 1 g dietary fiber, 167 mg sodium

Lemon Fluff

⬠ ⬠ ⬠ *Light and lemony, you can whip this recipe up without the whipped cream. We lightened up the original recipe by substituting evaporated skim milk for regular evaporated milk and diet gelatin for regular. Save 64 more calories by skipping the graham cracker crumbs. A good source of calcium with 100 milligrams, this is an excellent way to have your milk and eat a dessert too!*

1 (.3 oz.) pkg. diet lemon gelatin, prepared, partially set
1 cup evaporated skim milk, very cold
¼ cup lemon juice (1 lemon)
rind of 1 lemon, grated (2 tsp.)
⅔ cup sugar
1 cup graham cracker crumbs

Prepare gelatin. Whip milk and gradually add lemon juice, lemon rind and sugar. Fold partly set gelatin into whipped milk until mixed. Pour mixture over ½ cup crumbs in a 7"x10" dish and cover with remaining crumbs. When thoroughly set, cut in 8 squares. (Or omit crumbs and scoop into individual dessert glasses.) Garnish with thin slices of lemon.

Nutritional information per serving 158 calories, 4 g protein, 32 g carbohydrate, 1.6 g total fat, .5 g saturated fat, .6 g monounsaturated fat, .4 g polyunsaturated fat, 1 mg cholesterol, .5 g fiber, 130 mg sodium

Mocha Chocolate Soufflé

This "guilt-free" soufflé is a wonderful finale to a meal, yet low calorie! We used cocoa powder which is chocolate without the fat, and skim milk instead of whole milk, to create this elegant dessert. Very impressive when you have guests.

½ cup sugar
⅓ cup cocoa
1 tbs. cornstarch
1 cup skim milk
3 eggs, separated
1 tsp. vanilla extract
1 tsp. very strong coffee
¼ tsp. cream of tartar

Combine sugar, cocoa and cornstarch in the top of a double boiler; gradually add milk and stir. Cook over boiling water, stirring constantly until thickened. Beat egg yolks slightly. Gradually stir about ¼ of the hot mixture into yolks. Add egg yolks to remaining hot mixture, stirring constantly. Add vanilla and coffee. Cool to room temperature. Beat egg whites (at room temperature) with cream of tartar until stiff but not dry. Gently fold into chocolate mixture. Pour into individual custard cups or ramekins. Place in pan filled with about ½" of hot water. Bake at 350° for 25 to 30 minutes or until puffed. Serve immediately.

Nutritional information per serving   133 calories, 5 g protein, 22 g carbohydrate, 3.5 g total fat, 1.4 g saturated fat, 1.4 g monounsaturated fat, .4 g polyunsaturated fat, 105 mg cholesterol, 1 g dietary fiber, 56 mg sodium

Pear Sorbet

Servings: 4

🍐 ⭐ ▨ 🌾 *Pears and ginger are a great com-*
bination for this nutrition all-star
dessert. An added bonus is the 4 grams of dietary fiber.

1 (16 oz.) can sliced pears in light
 syrup, undrained
½ tsp. grated lemon rind
2 tbs. lemon juice
½ tsp. ground ginger
2 fresh unpeeled pears, thinly sliced
fresh mint leaves (optional)

Using the knife blade of the food processor, add undrained canned pears, lemon rind and lemon juice. Process pears until smooth; add ginger. Chill thoroughly and pour into freezer tray or an 8" square pan. Freeze until mixture is almost firm. Break mixture into pieces, place in processor bowl and process until light and fluffy but not thawed. Return to freezer tray and freeze until firm. To serve, let stand approximately 10 to 15 minutes before scooping with a spoon or ice cream scoop. Garnish each dish with ½ pear thinly sliced and fresh mint leaves, if desired.

Nutritional information per serving 117 calories, .6 g protein, 31 g carbohydrate, .4 g total fat, 0 g saturated fat, 0 g monounsaturated fat, .1 g polyunsaturated fat, 0 mg cholesterol, 4 g dietary fiber, 7 mg sodium

Bread Pudding with Brandy Sauce

Servings: 6

Bread pudding connoisseurs will give this light dessert a top rating. Quick, easy and low in fat, this is a great way to use leftover cinnamon raisin bread and also boost calcium intake.

    2 eggs, slightly beaten
    1/3 cup brown sugar, packed
    2 cups skim milk
    1 tsp. vanilla
    1/2 tsp. nutmeg
    4 slices cinnamon raisin bread, cubed

Combine eggs, brown sugar, milk, vanilla and nutmeg. Add bread cubes and stir. Let stand 5 minutes. Pour mixture into an 8" square baking dish which has been coated with nonstick cooking spray. Place baking dish in a larger pan which contains 1" of hot water. Bake at 350° for 35 minutes or until a knife inserted in the center comes out clean. Serve warm with hot **Brandy Sauce.**

Brandy Sauce

1 tbs. margarine
1 tbs. flour
½ cup boiling water
2 tbs. brown sugar
1 tbs. brandy (or sherry, whiskey or
  lemon juice)

Melt margarine and stir in flour until blended. Slowly add boiling water and brown sugar. Cook, stirring constantly, until bubbly. Add brandy. In a double boiler, cook mixture for 15 minutes.

Nutritional information per ½-cup serving with 1½ tbs. sauce   184 calories, 6.2 g protein, 30 g carbohydrate, 4.6 g total fat, 1.4 g saturated fat, 1.8 g monounsaturated fat, 1.1 g polyunsaturated fat, 71 mg cholesterol, .4 g dietary fiber, 155 mg sodium

Index

LOOK FOR THESE TITLES IN OUR
MATURE READER SERIES:

OVER 50 AND STILL COOKING!
Recipes for Good Health and Long Life

THE NUTRITION GAME:
The Right Moves if You're Over 50

THE ENCYCLOPEDIA OF GRANDPARENTING
Hundreds of Ideas to Entertain Your Grandchildren

DEALS & DISCOUNTS
If You're 50 or Older

START YOUR OWN BUSINESS
AFTER 50 — OR 60 — OR 70!
These People Did. Here's How:

I DARE YOU!
How to Stay Young Forever

THE BEGINNER'S ANCESTOR RESEARCH KIT
Start Climbing Your Family Tree

50 mg.

*Viagra - Pfizer   N.Y.U.
circulation*

*blocks enzyme   70%   helped.   diabetics
in penis   80%   50°-60%*

muscle relaxation

*helps
Physical or phys. co.
vascular problems.   — natural.*

Epileptics Nitrate users - Nitroglycerine should not ta